Home Health Care for Children Who Are Technology Dependent

ABOUT THE AUTHOR

Juanita W. Fleming, RN, PhD, FAAN, is Professor Emeritus at the University of Kentucky. During her tenure at the University she served in several roles, including Division Chair, Assistant and Associate Dean, Associate Vice Chancellor for Academic Affairs in the Medical Center, and Special Assistant to the President for Academic Affairs. She had Professorial rank in the Colleges of Nursing and Education. She received the baccalaureate degree in nursing with high honors, ranking in the top ten graduates of her class, from Hampton University, a Master of Arts from the University of Chicago, and as a recipient of the Mary Roberts Fellowship she studied Journalism and Human Development at the University of Maryland. Her PhD in Education of Exceptional Children and Psychology is from Catholic University of America. Her scholarly productivity is evidenced by her publications, grant activity, and invited presentations, as well as by her work as a reviewer and as a member of study sections, national committees, and councils. The many honors and awards she has received recognize her contributions in maternal child health and higher education. Among the honors she has received are memberships in the American Academy of Nursing and the Institute of Medicine. She is currently serving as the Interim Vice President for Academic Affairs at Kentucky State University. She is the mother of two sons, William and Robert, and the wife of Dr. William Fleming, Sr.

CONTRIBUTORS

Mary Barron, BSN, RN, is Research Nurse Coordinator, Family Practice, University of Kentucky Hospital, Lexington, Kentucky.

Nora F. Steele, DNS, RN, PNP, is Associate Professor and Educational Coordinator, Parent-Child Nursing, Charity-Delgado School of Nursing, New Orleans, Louisiana.

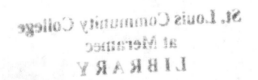

Home Health Care for Children Who Are Technology Dependent

Juanita W. Fleming, RN, PhD, FAAN

 Springer Publishing Company

Springer Publishing Company, Inc.
536 Broadway
New York, NY 10012-3955

Acquisitions Editor: Ruth Chasek
Production Editor: J. Hurkin-Torres
Cover design by Joanne Honigman

04 05 06 07 / 5 4 3 2 1

Library of Congress Cataloging-in-Publication Data

Fleming, Juanita W.
  Home health care for children who are technology dependent / Juanita W. Fleming.
      p. ; cm.
    Includes bibliographical references and index.
    ISBN 0-8261-2064-4
    1. Home care services. 2. Handicapped children—Services for. 3. Chronically ill children—Services for. 4. Medical technology. 1. Title.
    [DNLM: 1. Home Care Services—Child. 2. Caregivers—psychology. 3. Home Nursing—Child. 4. Medical Assistance. 5. Respite Care. 6. Social Support.
    WY 115 F597h 2004]
    RJ380.F545 2004
    362.198'92—dc22   2003059043

Printed in the United States of America by Integrated Book Technology.

Contents

Appendices

Foreword

D r. Juanita Fleming has completed a masterful document on children who are technology dependent. This book will help the reader view the world from the standpoint of the technology-dependent child and his or her family. Health care professionals of various backgrounds will find that this book will bring them up-to-date with the state of the art of the health care delivery system to these children and their families.

When one realizes there are more than 10 million children in the United States who depend on technology to sustain their lives, one understands the vital importance of this book. More and more children are being cared for in their homes, and nurses involved in home care need to be aware of the situation for the child and the family. While it is hoped that the child's medical condition is stable because of the wide range of complications that may occur with the various children and their illnesses, emergencies will need to be handled.

Dr. Fleming has provided the overview of the research evidence that is available on home health care of children who are technology dependent and their families. This information will help health-care professionals fulfill the needs of technology-dependent children and their families. She shares the information obtained from the major study that she conducted with colleagues around the United States. This information will challenge all who read the book to provide improved care.

The population of the children who are technology dependent and cared for at home is as follows: 45,000 need apnea monitoring. Renal dialysis is needed by up to 6,000 children. Ventilator assistance to children reaches more than 2,000, and over 8,000 children need prolonged intravenous drugs. As the years pass, more and more children will require these services. There will be new technologies that will become available in the home setting.

Dr. Fleming's background in childhood development is most useful as she reviews the literature as well as documents the interrelationships of children's health and family environment. Children with long-term health problems express themselves differently, and nurses need to be attuned to the differences based on age, sex, and developmental level.

Because of the complexity of care that technology-dependent children require, the mental health of the caregivers may be affected. Clues are given such as disheveled appearances, verbal response that is slow or halting, physical symptoms, and behavior. One needs to be alert to the stresses and rewards of providing this intensive care 24 hours a day, 7 days a week.

Because of the complexities facing these families, case management programs can be a lifesaver to the parents. Comprehensive services are required, and the case manager can work miracles for the families by providing the essential information needed for the various services.

Technology-dependent children may be a huge financial burden to families who do not have good health care coverage. States have different packages to help these families. The coverage can vary a great deal between states.

The appendix of this book includes very useful materials by providing the best practices for providing care to children who are technology dependent and their families.

In conclusion, this remarkable book by Dr. Fleming pulls together the essential content for all those who are concerned about technology-dependent children and their families. This valuable book would be excellent for undergraduate and graduate nurses. Practicing nurses who work with technology-dependent children will find this book a rich reference that will challenge them to improve their care to these children and families whether the child is in the hospital or at home.

IDA MARTINSON, RN, PhD, FAAN
PROFESSOR
UNIVERSITY OF CALIFORNIA–SAN FRANCISCO

Thomas, Quilla Turner, Barbara Wheeler, and Ann Young, who served as consulting coordinators. I thank Mr. James Wolfe, Ms. Annette Castle, Ms. Shirley Riggs, and Drs. Barbara Teague, Richard Kryscio, Barbara Kiernan, Marie Lobo, James Houghland, Sherry Shamansky, and Barbara Sachs for their roles in the study and their reports. From 1991 to 1995, individual members of this distinguished group of participants made more than 20 presentations of the study at conferences and meetings throughout the United States.

This is an opportunity to thank Dr. Gontran Lamberty and Dr. Woodie Kessel for their support and their commitment to improving the lives of all children through research and practice. This commitment was reflected during and following the study. I am grateful to Dr. Charles T. Wethington, Jr., President Emeritus, University of Kentucky, for his understanding and for allowing me to complete this research study and share information from it, when he hired me as Special Assistant for Academic Affairs, a position I held from February 1991 to June 2001 and to Dr. Angela McBride, for encouraging me to prepare this book.

I am indebted to Dr. Ida Martinson, whose seminal work on home care of dying children has made a unique contribution to their care, for her review of the entire manuscript, and for the foreword that she has so eloquently written. My deepest thanks to Dr. Laura Hayman, an outstanding pediatric nurse educator, for her review of the chapters dealing with evidence and best practice, and to Dr. Kathryn Barnard, another outstanding educator, researcher, and administrator, for the information she provided on NCAST. Her stellar work has made and continues to make a valuable contribution in the care of young children. Thanks to Dr. Lynne Hall, Assistant Dean for Doctoral Education and Research in the College of Nursing, University of Kentucky, whose brilliance and dedication to nursing research is readily apparent, for assigning Ms. Mary Barron as a graduate assistant to work with me in conducting a follow-up study of the participating caregivers of children who were technology dependent in the study noted above. Ms Barron was tenacious in trying to locate the parental caregivers, and her dedication to follow through on every lead is greatly appreciated. Many of the citations in the book are the result of CINAHL, MEDLINE, psychological and sociological literature, and other databases obtained by Ms. Gail O'Malley. I am deeply indebted to her for this assistance, and for the multiple books and articles she obtained for my use. Finally, I thank Ms. Deborah Sparkman for her dedicated efforts in doing the word processing for the manuscript and preparing it for the publisher; Ms. Ruth Chasek, Nursing Editor, for her feedback, guidance, and responsiveness to queries made; and my husband, Dr. William Fleming, for his patience and support while I worked on this manuscript.

Acknowledgments

The stimulus for this book is my abiding interest in ensuring that as the health care environment continues to change in this twenty-first century, the care of families and their children who are dependent on technology and home care remains visible and recognized as an important dimension of health care. My interest in the plight of these children and their families started years ago when as a parent–child faculty member of students in a graduate program I learned that some families caring for children in their home were ineligible for Supplemental Security Income (SSI) to assist them with care in spite of documentation they provided. From a social-psychological perspective, these children and their families appeared invisible, powerless to get consideration for the plight in which they found themselves. On the one hand, medical knowledge had kept these children alive and was meeting their physiological needs using medical devices, but from a social perspective, they were neglected and treated callously in many respects, like some other minority groups in the society at times.

It was an honor and a privilege to serve as a member of the work group selected to develop more individualized criteria as a result of the Supreme Court's decision in the Brian Zebley case. (See "Policy Issues" on page 224 for Zebley case discussion.) The service given was one of the activities that added value to my career. The opportunity to testify before the U.S. Congress on behalf of the American Nurses Association about this population group was of great significance to me and exemplifies the profession of nursing's commitment to children who are technology dependent.

I would like to express special gratitude for receipt of the competitive grant MCJ-210577 from the Maternal and Child Health Program (Title V, Social Security Act) Health Resources and Services Administration, Department of Health and Human Services, which supported a national research study of technology-dependent children and their families and for the extraordinary and talented individuals who worked diligently to ensure that the study was implemented. They were Drs. Mary Challela, Joanne Eland, Renata Hornick, Phyllis Johnson, Ida Martinson, Donna Nativio, Kathleen Nokes, Irene Riddle, Nora Steele, Katherine Sudela, Robin

Part I

Overview

Chapter 1

Introduction

Mary Barron and Juanita Fleming

C hildren who are technology dependent are those who need both a surviving medical device to compensate for loss of a vital body function and ongoing nursing care to avert death or further disability. Technological advances in medical care have allowed many children to survive and recover from catastrophic illness, traumatic injuries, and both acquired and congenital health problems. Along with these technological advances, children need compassionate adults to care for them day to day for survival. These compassionate adults are family members guided by health care professionals. This chapter will consider suggestions for health professionals based on the current literature, my study of 898 technology-dependent children, and a recently completed follow-up study to assist these children and their families with home care. It will also highlight suggestions to health care professionals from families of older technology-dependent children. Having met the challenges of caring for infants of technology-dependent newborns, some parents share their thoughts and feelings about the services of health care professionals.

Please note that there is a very limited amount of research that has been published on this topic, and for this reason the word "current" is used to cover a longer period of time than readers are accustomed to in other health care specialties.

A GREATER POPULATION OF TECHNOLOGY-DEPENDENT CHILDREN IN HOME CARE WITH MULTIPLE NEEDS

Numerous studies have revealed that families of technology-dependent children experience increased stress emotionally, physically, psychologically, and financially (Cohen & Warren, 1985; Hobbs, Perrin, Ireys, Moyni-han, & Shayne, 1984; Odnoha, 1986; Stullenberger, Norris, Edgil, & Prosser, 1987). Emotionally, caregivers experience denial, anger, depression, chronic sorrow, and loss of freedom (Murphy, 1991). The "perfect, normal child" has been lost. Physically, the demands of caring for a dependent child are often exhausting. Not only is there the physical care involved with a child who may be immobile, but there is also the often 24-hour care with little or no time for rest, and the continued visits with therapists, doctors, home health providers, and others. Psychologically, in the case of an infant, these caregivers not only deal with the arrival of a newborn but also the arrival of a newborn who is medically fragile. This challenges the new parents' feelings of competency and deepens concerns for the infant's well-being (Miller & Myers-Walls, 1983; Sollie & Miller, 1980; Ventura, 1987).

As if these stresses are not enough for the caregiver to deal with, the financial burden of caring for a technology-dependent infant in the home must be addressed. Because of hospitals' cost containment efforts and changing social norms, the numbers of chronically ill and/or technology-dependent children being released from institutional care are rising. Sustaining children who need medical technology can be expensive, depending on the extent of the need and the type of equipment required (Parette, 1993). Third-party payers' answer to this rising cost is to discharge these children from hospitals earlier and depend on home caregivers (O'Connor, Plaats, & Betz, 1992). Although home care is supposedly less costly than hospital care, there are indicators that we have only shifted this financial burden to the families of these children. Fleming and colleagues (1994) discovered in their study of the impact of technology-dependent children on their families (described in chapter 4) that it is especially difficult when parents are young, unemployed, have limited education, and are isolated geographically. Spalding and McKeever (1998) relate that in their study of mothers of children with gastrostomy tube dependence, out of eight unemployed mothers interviewed, six reported that they could not work because they had "full-time jobs" caring for their children with disabilities. We have simply transferred the financial burden to individuals who we know will be unable to meet the costs of caring for these children.

NURSING IMPLICATIONS

Meeting the needs of a child who is dependent on medical technology often involves various types of health care providers. Personnel involved in the care of one child may include specialty physicians, physical and/or occupational therapists, speech therapists, nutritionists, special educators and other school personnel, psychologists, social workers, and nurses. This multidisciplinary team is often involved in the hospital, home, community, and/or school environment (Ahmann & Lierman, 1992). Because of the potential for error with so many team players and settings in the management of these children, experts in this area have been suggesting nurse case management for these families (Ahmann & Lierman, 1992; Fleming et al., 1994).

In 1992, Ahmann and Lierman suggested nurse case management for technology-dependent children and their families that would involve the development and routine evaluation of an overall care plan that involves all the players of the multidisciplinary team. This care plan would provide a mechanism by which family members and providers would become aware of their responsibilities for the care of the child, while monitoring the provision of the services rendered by the health care professionals for quality of care and duplication of services. This care plan would also provide a vehicle through which the family and providers could communicate with one another, and providers could communicate with each other as needed (Ahmann & Lipsi, 1991; Gittler, 1988).

Fleming and colleagues (1994) suggest that the case management begin in the hospital during the child's acute episode. It should begin with the assurance that the caregivers have received adequate education and training on the proper use of their child's support equipment. In a study looking at the mood states, family functioning, and support systems of mothers with infants on apnea monitors, Knecht (1991) supports the concept of early case management in the hospital. This study revealed that during the transition of a technology-dependent child into the home care setting, the onset and termination of technological support was felt by mothers to be the most threatening to normal family functioning. The onset and termination of technological support traditionally coincide with hospitalization, making early case management one of the most appealing interventions for these families.

In situations where nurse case management is not feasible for these families, Stephenson (1999) has suggested that health care professionals refer the child and his/her family to the appropriate state comprehensive early intervention services. All states are required to maintain comprehensive early intervention programs for developmentally delayed children. Each child will be assigned a coordinator who, through the assessment of family demands, coping, and well-being, will develop a plan of care designed to meet individual family needs.

Anticipatory guidance on caregiving at home has also reached the fore-front in the last few years. McCaleb and Luther (1996) have urged nurses to help families assess their strengths and weaknesses before the release of their child from the hospital. This will enable the family to anticipate the coping patterns and support needed before going home with the child. Although each family is unique in its characteristics, some factors, such as depression, sorrow, fatigue, and frustration, eventually become evident in almost all families caring for technology-dependent children (Stephenson, 1999).

Exhaustion from the intensive care of a dependent child fosters family dysfunction, eventually leading to less focused care for the child. As Stephenson (1999) has shared, the progress of an infant often depends on the family's ability to secure medical assistance, and, likewise, the infant's progress affects the family interactions. As one of these fails, the other must be stronger to compensate. But how can caregivers be strong if they are physically and emotionally exhausted from the long hours of rendering care? Most researchers feel that the answer to this problem is respite care (Fleming et al., 1994; O'Connor, Plaats, & Betz, 1992; Spalding & McKeever, 1998; Teague et al., 1993). In an effort to prevent the emotional, physical, psychological, and financial exhaustion of caregivers, respite care is designed as a support service to temporarily relieve the caregiver from the responsibilities of caring for the technology-dependent child (Cohen & Warren, 1985; Odnoha, 1986).

To be beneficial, health care professionals must be alert to the signs of respite care need. Evidence of parents becoming overwhelmed or exhausted can include the following: (1) comments about their lack of time to do anything other than care for their technology-dependent child, (2) inability to spend time with other children or mate, (3) physical signs, such as the parent appearing disheveled, (4) low energy level or hyperactive signs of anxiety (fatigue, irritability, and impatience), (5) behavioral problems in the children who are not technology dependent, and/or (6) marital problems, and so forth. Recognition of these warning signs should not only prompt a referral of the family to respite care but also assist the family to find specific, appropriate referral agencies for their situation. O'Connor et al. (1992) note that health care workers must aid the family in making this connection and suggest that respite care agencies should use the available resource of parents as trainers for new respite caregivers for their child.

Researchers have also found that not only is it vital to monitor family and caregiver function, but we must also monitor the developmental stages of these children. Although these children experience periods of medical instability, they progress through the same developmental stages as healthy children. Through assessment, planning, and collaboration with parents and other health care providers, nurses play a vital role in helping these children and families make the transition through the developmental stages (Ahmann & Lierman, 1992). Looking at the self-enabling abilities of young ventilator-dependent people, Noyes (2000) was able to express these children's status most effectively by advising health care professionals that these children are not passive recipients of care but active participants in life. Those involved in her study expressed the wish not to be treated simply as a medical case, but as a developing young person with wider social needs. Apperiesto et al. (2002) substantiate the belief that home care of children requiring ventilatory support improves their outcomes and results in cost saving. They report on 46 children with chronic respiratory failure who were included in a home care program in Rome. Thirty-seven children lived at home and four of them improved enough that it was possible to remove the tracheostomy tube. Their oldest patient has now been on mechanical ventilation at home for 15 years.

Finally, nurses and other health care professionals have been urged to advocate for this population of children being cared for in their home (Fleming et al., 1994). Overburdened families cannot do this advocating alone. Health care providers must work with these families to seek out what is best for each child. The most important role that nurses can fill in helping these children is to guide their families to the best possible services available, thereby leading to a fulfilling lifestyle for technology-dependent children and their families.

HOW WELL ARE WE DOING IN FULFILLING THE NEEDS OF THESE CHILDREN AND THEIR FAMILIES?

In an effort to assess how some of these families were doing several years after the implementation of a study conducted by Fleming et al. (1994), an attempt was made to contact 848 primary caregivers of technology-dependent children ages 3 months to 19 years being cared for at home who participated in the study of families receiving both public and private services in 13 cities, described later in this book. One of the purposes of the original study was to indicate the impact on the families of four categories or groups of technology-dependent children (those requiring: ventilator assistance, parenteral nutrition or prolonged intravenous drugs, device-based respiratory or nutritional support, or apnea monitoring, renal dialysis or other device-assisted nursing). Random samples of 42 of these families were contacted by telephone in 1999–2000 to see how the children were doing after a time lapse of approximately six years and to look at the concerns of parents and caregivers regarding their child and the services of the health care industry. At the end of the telephone interview, the caregivers were asked to give the interviewer any suggestions, concerns, or opinions regarding their child, family, or technology-dependent children in general. These suggestions, concerns, and opinions will be discussed.

At the time of interview, the children ranged from 7 to 18 years of age. Five of them had died since the first interview with the caregiver, in 1993–1994. Of the 37 caregivers interviewed, only a few of these indicated that the children currently required the assistance of a technology device. Ten of the caregivers reported that their child's condition still required the assistance of health care professionals in the home. These professionals included nine nurses and one behavioral therapist. The amount of time these health care professionals spent in the home varied from occasional respite care to 112 hours of nursing time per week. When the interviewees were asked about their child's academic, behavioral, and social development, most were very pleased to say that despite the child's current or past use of technological devices for health care, their child's developmental functioning in these areas was about average for children of the same age. Academically, ten children were ranked as below average, 18 as about average, and 9 as more advanced than other children of the same age. Behaviorally and socially, 11 children were ranked as below average, 18 as about average, and 8 as more advanced.

The suggestions, concerns, and opinions varied among the group. Some of the caregivers interviewed offered no opinions, but most did and were eager to speak to someone who was advocating for this group of children. Because the majority of these children had become nondependent on medical technology, the most prevailing emotions from caregivers were relief and great pride in their child for physical, academic, behavioral, and social success.

However, some of these parents were still dealing with the daily care of a technology-dependent child and appreciated the opportunity to share their ideas and opinions with someone in the health care system. The prevailing comment from this group was the need for more nursing and other respite workers in the home setting. Many times these parents are caring for siblings of the dependent child also. Efforts by the caregivers to make family life as "normal" and functional as possible results in exhaustion. The effect that this exhaustion has on caregivers is best summed up by this mother:

> I am so thankful for the number of nursing hours that we receive each week because I know that it is more than many families receive, but it still is just not enough. While my child is in school, I am able to function with the amount of nursing hours that we get because he also gets nursing hours from the school system during school hours. This lets us save our hours from the home health agency for after school and on weekends. When school is not open, we lose the 8 hours per day that the school provides. It makes even a trip to the grocery store a struggle. Summer vacation begins next week and I know that I am not ready for this again yet.

Caregivers emphasize their thankfulness for the nursing hours that they have but declare that the number one thing that their family could use now would be more respite hours. One mother even suggested that local universities provide training for nursing students by allowing them to provide respite care for families of technology-dependent children. These families did not ask for more funding to be allotted for additional nursing time. They know that funding is limited. They were willing to make suggestions that would not cost the system additional money, such as the services of nursing students.

Other caregivers wanted to give advice to parents who were facing the task of caring for a technology-dependent child for the first time. One mother shared that she would like parents/guardians to acknowledge that while health care professionals are vital in the medical care of their child, parents are the most reliable judges of what their child can and cannot accomplish. This same mother related, "If we had listened to the health care system about what our son would and would not be able to do in the future, he would not be where he is today." She expressed gratitude for what the medical professionals had been able to do for her child but said that it could not have been accomplished without parents or guardians.

Although the majority of the families interviewed had graduated from the stage of technological dependence and were raising healthy, normal children, we still need to serve the families that continue to provide in-home care to technology-dependent children in late childhood. It seems that these families have emerged from the early phases of shock, sorrow, and acceptance. They are now in a different stage of development and what resounds from them is the need for more respite care. Anticipatory guidance for bringing a technology-dependent newborn home from the hospital and coordination of services are two early tasks to be done by these families and health professionals. Now we need to move on to the next phase of advocating for more respite care services for them. As Fleming et al. outlined in 1994, it is our responsibility as professional caregivers to advocate for this group of special needs children. This is one stage of development these families can never navigate alone. Respite care is greatly needed whether the child is 2 days or 18 years old.

After several years of home care, one may wonder if all of the families studied were able to care for a special needs child and keep their family together and functioning well. This is a question that must be left unanswered. In attempting to complete these 42 parent/guardian interviews, we were unable to contact 121 others due to the reported telephone number being disconnected. An additional 40 other children were no longer residing at the location of the telephone number listed. Two other children had been removed form the listed foster care home and were not able to be located. Further steps taken to locate these children and to determine their well-being included the contact of operators for area code changes and the search for parents via the World Wide Web.

One can only speculate as to the well-being of these children today. Has the physical, emotional, and financial burden of the care of a special needs child resulted in transient behavior of these families? Have we as health care professionals sufficiently supported these families in their communities, or have they moved on to other communities for support? Where are these children today and are they doing as well as the families that completed interviews? Are they experiencing the same frustration at the lack of respite care as those we interviewed? Through the praise it is clear that we are advocating for these children; yet we must continue to advocate for them as they grow into early and late childhood.

Consistent technological advances in medical care have resulted in a growing number of children surviving and/or recovering from catastrophic illness, traumatic injuries and both acquired and congenital health problems (Feinberg, 1985). The movement of complex medical care into the home has met with a level of success. Martinson (1976) is one of the few nurses who conducted the early research on home care for children. Home care was viewed, when she conducted her research and now, as one segment of the continuum of progressive patient care. It was seen as an alternative to hospitalization for dying children. Today hospice care has taken up the gauntlet of providing care in the home to dying individuals. Martinson (1976) provided an enlightened perspective on the family and professionals involved in home care of the dying. The role of the nurse and the technical aspects of care are presented in her work. Cost of home care for dying children and the methods used to determine costs were also studied.

Moldow, Armstrong, Henry, and Martinson (1982) did a comparison of costs for comfort care during the final days of the life of children dying of cancer who were being treated at home and those being treated in the hospital. Depending on what specifically was being compared, the hospital care cost about 22% to 207% more than home care. If the child is medically stable, it is likely that the cost of medical and nursing care will be less expensive if care is provided in the home than it will be if care is provided in the hospital. The costs, however, to the family in terms of other factors may not be measured in terms of money alone.

New technologies have affected nursing dramatically in the last four decades and will continue to do so. Nursing practice is dependent on (1) having some conceptualization of the characteristics of the children who are technology-dependent and their families, (2) enhancement of their knowledge and relevant nursing skills in the effective and appropriate use of the technologies, and (3) recognition that many parents prefer home care to a hospital stay for their children who are technology-dependent and that in order to provide effective home care of high quality the family will need:

- adequate training and preparation
- appropriate and well-maintained equipment
- adequate social and psychological support services
- proper transportation
- availability in the community of emergency facilities
- competent case management service
- high quality respite care service

LIMITATIONS AND IMPLICATIONS OF STUDIES FOR NURSING PRACTICE

Strengthening the family appears to be a critical factor in the provision of care for the child who is technology dependent and receiving care at home. Smith (1991) notes that medical advances alone cannot provide all of the solutions to caring for these children. Family stress and coping are factors that are essential to consider in the provision of home care to children who are technology dependent. Nursing assessment and interventions begin before the child is discharged from the hospital to home. Assessment is important, as well as reassessment as needed. Health care providers should initially obtain a family history, which should include financial information. McCoy and Votroubek (1990) delineate several financial considerations that need to be addressed before the child is placed in home care. Home care needs should be anticipated at the time of hospitalization, and home care benefits should be determined early in the child's hospitalization. Choosing a home care agency and taking advantage of the various funding programs available to help finance home care should be done. Benefits should be checked thoroughly when negotiating insurance coverage. It is suggested that families be cost conscious, especially with suppliers and equipment. Documentation is essential in paying for home care services.

Planning with the family and setting goals is an important aspect of assessment. Cultural aspects of care should be considered and included in plans of care. Maintaining ongoing dialogue with the family, clarifying expectations, identifying support services, and explaining situations or procedures as needed are other important dimensions of strengthening the family and providing quality care.

Transmitting knowledge about therapeutic techniques to caregivers of technology-dependent children is another important dimension of strengthening the family. Caregivers will not be able to assume responsibility for aspects of care unless they are taught. Strickling (1993) indicated the importance of education for home care consumers, noting the following as important: clear instruction, including good quality, illustrated teaching materials; timeliness of scheduled visits; consistency of staff; trust in the staff; concern, listening, and attention; and the tailoring of the teaching plan to the capability, readiness, and cultural preferences of the family. The health care provider should observe carefully and initiate changes as needed and intervene when appropriate. Care should be provided as needed for specific health problems when they arise. A goal for the family and the child is the prevention of rehospitalization, the promotion and maintenance of optimal development, and the physical and emotional functioning of the child and his/her family. Considering that a variety of services may be needed to achieve the goals, the nurse is likely to be the constant professional and may be expected to

- coordinate care
- have knowledge about pathophysiology of disease processes and intervention strategies that are appropriate to functioning levels
- have assessment skills
- have knowledge of equipment
- understand normal growth and development of the child

- understand family development
- have interpersonal and communication skills
- have knowledge of community resources
- have knowledge of financial resources

The theoretical basis for dependent health care is not as well developed as it should be. Taylor, Renpenning, Neuman, and Hart (2001) indicate that there are still elements of theory that need further development, such as specifying the enabling abilities of the dependent care agency and verifying and formalizing the various elements presented.

Family-centered care seems basic to the best practices for these children. Nurses recognize that families are intricately involved and cannot be effectively worked with if all members are not considered. The importance of case management for the child may be the role of the parent, the role of the nurse, or both. There is an extensive base of literature on case management and its relevance to providing care (Lamb, 1995). The notion of working with caregivers as partners and delivering family-centered care requires some unique skills on the part of the nurse.

Supporting families is an involved process and may not be easy to implement because of family dynamics. Dunst, Trivette, Starnes, Hamby, and Gordon (1993) note six basic principles of the family support movement that have been extracted from the literature:

1. Family support programs aim to integrate families into the mainstream to enhance a sense of community.
2. Family support programs mobilize resources and support, working to address the broad-based needs of families in addition to specific child-focused concerns.
3. Family support programs encourage shared responsibility and collaboration, ensure that professionals treat families like partners, and strengthen and protect the integrity of the family unit.
4. Family support programs encourage stable and healthy relations.
5. Family support systems operate according to enabling and empowering principles that enhance and promote competence of the family and individual family members. These principles create opportunities for family members to acquire knowledge, skills, and capacities so that they may become more capable and competent.
6. Family support systems follow a proactive human service approach, which is service-based and designed to meet the specific needs of the individual family.

It is important that those providing a support program function in a realistic manner, recognize the multifaceted nature of social support, and understand that most of the research done has focused on the short-term consequences that such support has for coping with life events. The long-term consequences of healthy functioning have remained largely unexplored (Pierce, Sarason, Sarason, Joseph, & Henderson, 1996).

Financial reimbursement for home health care continues to be an issue that needs to be addressed, as there seem to be limited funds to meet the needs of families who care for technology-dependent children in the home. This is essentially a policy matter that has implications for home care. Any policy issue implemented for cost efficiency must also provide for quality monitoring and assurance.

Managed care does not appear to be going away. In spite of its limitations and negatives, there are positive aspects, such as the intent to prevent illness when possible and to provide for people with ill health across the continuum of care. It has a promise for providing various integrated services required by individuals, such as children who are technology dependent. The expectation is that high-quality care is delivered and that it responds to the patient's needs and preferences. The expectation reflects the importance of the consumer. Health professionals who have been the high priests and priestesses not only will have to develop skills and competencies that reflect concerns about cost containment, efficiency, and patient satisfaction but also will need to consider the emphasis on evidence-based practice.

Maurano (1994) expects the home care market for children to continue to grow. By all measures, there will be even greater numbers of people affected by chronic conditions. She projects that there will be 39 million people with a chronic condition that causes limitation in their ability to go to school, to work, or to live independently. While many of these individuals will be elderly, a large number of them will be children under 19 years of age. In 1994 about one in every 15 children had activity-limiting chronic conditions (Institute for Health and Aging, 1996). As Maurano (1994) noted, an increased number of children are surviving because of medical technology. Haffner and Schurman (2001) note that improvements in the provision of oxygen, mechanical ventilation, tracheostomy care, enteral and parenteral nutrition, and dialysis have expanded the population of technology-dependent children. Reports of the increase in the numbers of technology-dependent children living at home in other countries and the costs for caring for them (Glendinning, Kirk, Guiffrida, & Lawton, 2001; Hammer, 2000) indicate that the concern for this population of children is not unique to the United States. The implication for the increase is this: Where will the funds come from to provide the resources and care that will be needed for this growing population group? Integrated services must be provided for children who are technology dependent and their families.

Beck, Hammond-Cordero, and Poole (1994) note the importance of one community's service approach to meet the needs of this population group that can be replicated in other communities. The provision of culturally competent health care also is an essential.

Quality of care from the perspective of life-saving, life-sustaining, and life-enhancing dimensions for children who are technology dependent and cared for at home are considerations for advocacy of these children and their families. The Home Care Bill of Rights indicates that home care consumers (clients) have a right to dignity and respect, decision making, financial information, and the highest quality of care. It has been our experience to encounter many health professionals who are committed and willing to be accountable for assuring that this population group, like others in the health care system, receives the highest quality of care available. They recognize that no solutions are permanent because as these children mature and grow, they are likely to become more independent or have different problems and adjustments to make, as will their families. The care of children, regardless of their condition, is dynamic because of the developmental expectations for them.

CONCLUSIONS

Children who are technology dependent and cared for in their homes by their families are a small but growing subset of a disabled, often chronically ill population who rely on life-sustaining medical devices and who otherwise would require complex hospital nursing care. Advances in medical technology are responsible for the survival of many of these children. This group of children ranges from those requiring the continuous assistance of a device and a highly trained caregiver to those requiring less frequent treatment and intermittent nursing care.

The nurse should observe and initiate changes as needed, intervene when appropriate, provide nursing care for specific health problems as they arise, and have as goals the prevention of rehospitalization and the promotion and maintenance of optimal developmental, physical, and emotional functioning of the child and his/her family.

Despite the stress that families encounter and the complexities they face, many are satisfied with the care their children receive and want to keep them at home. Predictors of caregiver and family stress are highlighted in Table 1.1.

Wegener and Aday (1989), in discussing home care for ventilator-assisted children, identify three categorical predictors of caregiver and family stress (see Table 1.1). The authors note that these predictors are not only useful as a profile identifying individual families at risk of high stress levels but also provide guidance for policies and programs to reduce stress on such families. They further delineate policy and programmatic implications of these predictors. The observations of Wegener and Aday

TABLE 1.1   Predictors of Caregiver and Family Stress Identified by Wegener and Aday

Family Finances

- Family assessment that finances are a serious problem for them.
- Family identification of a large number of out-of-pocket expenses incurred during the child's initial hospitalization (for example, expenses for transportation, lost income from work, extra telephone costs, parking, etc.).

Social and Physical Environment

- Families whose child has recently been discharged from the acute care setting, which may indicate some degree of initial unfamiliarity and adjustment required by families.
- Family living arrangements that include large numbers of extended family members (for example, grandparents, aunts, uncles, etc.).

Comprehensiveness of Child's Discharge Plan

- Families without a designated nurse case manager at discharge (family may have had another health care professional or no person designated as case manager).
- Families whose child's discharge planning included fewer elements of the guidelines established by the American Academy of Pediatrics' (AAP's) Ad Hoc Task Forces on Home Care of Chronically Ill Infants and Children.
- Families whose children had been seen by a greater number of physicians—children with primary diagnoses or additional conditions that required a number of specialists or families whose children were followed by a resident in a tertiary care institute and thus experienced the effect of rotations of individual doctors on and off cases (a lack of continuity of care).

Wegener, D. H., & Aday, L. A. (1989). Home care of ventilator assisted children: Predicting family stress. *Pediatric Nursing, 15*(4), 375.

seem appropriate for any family that has a child who is technology dependent and cared for in the home.

More advances in technology and changes in governmental policies may be expected as the technologies become available for use. Health care professionals will become more aware of the various needs of these children and their families. Based on the research available to date, families need information, psychosocial support, and assistance with the technology to meet the child's physiological, psychosocial, and developmental needs.

The lack of adequate funding has been a major impediment to successful home care and to some extent still is. In 1987, the Surgeon General (Koop, 1987) noted that "inadequate insurance, limitations on benefits, deductibles, co-payments, lack of coverage of certain types of services and limits on maximum lifetime benefits all place significant hardships on families caring for children with special health care needs" (p. 29). The State Child Health Insurance Program (SCHIP 2000) should be helpful.

The collaborative education positions taken to enhance patient safety by the Council on Graduate Medical Education and the National Advisory Council on Nurse Education and Practice will also benefit families and children who are technology dependent (Collaborative Education to Ensure Patient Safety, 2000). Interdisciplinary teams in the transmission of knowledge, conduct of research, and provision of care for this unique group of children are worthy of consideration because of the multiple types of services many of these children need.

Most of the studies of technology-dependent children use a descriptive approach. As will be noted in other parts of this book, other types of research are needed. Research is needed to enhance evidence-based practice. It will provide a knowledge base on which to make decisions, aid with the art and science of practice, and help provide better care to patients without having to rely on trial and error, tradition and authority, just plain common sense, inspiration, or intuition. Using educationally sound principles based on scientifically tested and reliable approaches provides a conceptual or theoretical foundation for practice.

We live in an age that depends increasingly on the intelligence, competence, imaginativeness, industriousness, and creativity of health care workers. There are those who indicate that knowledge is power. My premise is it is only power when we know what to do, when to do it, where to do it, on whom to do it, how to do it, and why we are doing it. To ensure that professional nursing continues to be a viable force in the health care arena, innovative research is a must. It is the only sure way to assure public and policy makers that nurses make a valuable contribution to health care.

REFERENCES

Ahmann, E., & Lierman, D. (1992). Promoting normal development in technology-dependent children: An introduction to issues. *Pediatric Nursing, 18*(2), 143–148.

Ahmann, E., & Lipsi, K. A. (1991). Early intervention for technology-dependent infants and young children. *Infants and Young Children, 3*(4), 67–77.

Appierto, L., Cori, M., Bianchi, R., Onofri, A., Catena, S., Ferrari, M., & Villani, A. (2002). Home care for chronic respiratory failure in children: 15 years experience. *Paediatric Anaesthesia, 12*(4), 345–350.

Beck, L. R., Hammond-Cordero, M., & Poole, J. (1994). Integrated services for children who are medically fragile and technology dependent. *Infants and Young Children, 6*(3), 75–83.

Betz, C. L. (1985). The pediatric patient: Strategies for improving interactions. *Home Health Care Nurse, 3*(4), 11–17.

Cohen, S., & Warren, R. (1985). Respite care. *Rehabilitation Literature, 46,* 66–71.

Collaborative Education to Ensure Patient Safety. (2000). Graduate Council on Medical Education and the National Advisory Council on Nurse Education and Practice.

Cowart, M. E. (1985). Policy issues: Financial reimbursement for home care. *Family and Community Health, 8*(2), 1–10.

Dunst, C. J., Trivette, C. M., Starnes, A. L., Hamby, D. W., & Gordon, N. J. (1993). Families, disability and empowerment. In G. H. S. Singer & E. L. Powers (Eds.), *Families, disabilities and empowerment* (pp. 89–118). Baltimore, MD: Paul H. Brooks.

Fleming, J. (1985). Maternal-child nursing in the decade ahead. *American Journal of Maternal-Child Nursing, 10,* 369–370, 374, 376.

Fleming, J., Challela, M., Eland, J., Hornick, R., Johnson, P., Martinson, I., Nativio, D., Nokes, K., Riddle, I., Steele, N., Sudela, K., Thomas, R., Turner, Q., Wheeler, B., & Young, A. (1994). Impact on the family of children who are technology dependent and cared for in the home. *Pediatric Nursing, 20*(4), 379–388.

Foster, R. (1989). Principles and strategies of home care. In R. Foster, M. Hunsberger, & J. J. T. Anderson (Eds.), *Family centered nursing care of children* (pp. 995–1013).

Gittler, J. (1988). Case management for children with special health needs. In H. M. Wallace, G. Ryan, & A. C. Oglesby (Eds.), *Maternal and child health practices* (3rd ed., pp. 659–666). Oakland, CA: Third Party.

Glendinning, C., Kirk, S., Guiffrida, A., & Lawton, D. (2001). Technology dependent children in the community: Definitions, numbers and costs. *Child-care Health and Development, 27*(4), 321–324.

Haffner, J. C., & Schurman, S. J. (2001). The technology dependent child. *Pediatric Clinics of North America, 48*(3), 751–764.

Hammer, J. (2000). Home mechanical ventilation in children. *Schweizerische-Medizinische-Wochenschrift, 130*(49), 1894–1902.

Hobbs, N., Perrin, J., Ireys, H. T., Moynihan, L., & Shayne, M. (1984). Chronically ill children in America. *Rehabilitation Literature, 45,* 206–213.

Kaufman, J., & Hardy-Ribakow, D. (1988). Home care: A model of a comprehensive approach for technology assisted chronically ill children. *Journal of Pediatric Nursing,* 2(4), 244–249.

Knecht, L. D. (1991). Home apnea monitoring: Mother's mood states, family functioning, and support systems. *Public Health Nursing, 8,* 154–160.

Koop, C. E. (1987). *Surgeon General's report on children with special care needs: Commitment to family-centered, community-based, coordinated care.* Rockville, MD: U.S. Department of Health and Human Services. Public Health Service.

Lamb, G. S. (1995). Case management. In J. J. Fitzpatrick & J. S. Stevenson (Eds.), *Annual Review of Nursing Research, 13,* 117–136.

Maurano, L. W. (1994). Community and home care. In C. L. Betz, M. Hunsberger, & S. T. Wright (Eds.), *Family-centered nursing care of children* (pp. 782–803). Philadelphia: W. B. Saunders.

McCaleb, A., & Luther, L. S. (1996). Characteristics and coping patterns of families with infants on home apnea monitoring. *Issues in Comprehensive Pediatric Nursing,* 19, 81–92.

McCoy, P., & Votroubek, W. L. (Eds.). (1990). *Pediatric home care: A comprehensive approach.* Rockville, MD: Aspen.

Miller, B. C., & Myers-Walls, J. (1983). Parenthood: Stressors and coping strategies. In H. I. McCubbin & C. R. Figley (Eds.), *Stress and the family: Vol 1: Coping with normative transitions.* New York: Brunner/Mazel.

Murphy, K. (1991). Stress and coping in home care: A study of families. In J. J. Hochstadt & P. Yost (Eds.), *The medically complex child* (pp. 287–302). New York: Harwood Academic Publishers.

Noyes, J. (2000). Enabling young "ventilator-dependent" people to express their views and experiences of their care in hospital. *Journal of Advanced Nursing, 31*(5), 1206–1215.

O'Connor, P., Plaats, S. V., & Betz, C. L. (1992). Respite care services to caretakers of chronically ill children in California. *Journal of Pediatric Nursing, 7*(4), 269–275.

Odnoha, C. (1986). Respite program for families of chronically ill children. *Caring,* 5, 20–24.

Parette, H. P., Jr. (1993). High-risk infant case management and assistive technology: Funding and family enabling perspectives. *Maternal-Child Nursing Journal, 21,* 53–64.

Pierce, G. R., Sarason, B. R., Sarason, I. G., Joseph, H. J., & Henderson, C. A. (1996). Conceptualizing and assessing social support in the context of the family. In G. R. Pierce, B. R. Sarason, & I. G. Sarason (Eds.), *Handbook of social support and the family* (pp. 3–23). New York: Plenum.

Smith, S. J. (1991). Promoting family adaptation to the at-home care of the technology-dependent child. *Issues in Comprehensive Pediatric Nursing, 14,* 249–258.

Sollie, D. L., & Miller, B. C. (1980). The transition to parenthood: A critical time for building family strengths. In J. Stennett, B. Chesser, J. DeFrain, & P. Knaub (Eds.), *Family strengths: Positive model for family life.* Lincoln: University of Nebraska Press.

Spalding, K., & McKeever, P. (1998). Mothers' experiences caring for children with disabilities who require a gastrostomy tube. *Journal of Pediatric Nursing, 13*(4), 234–243.

Stephenson, C. (1999). Well-being of families with healthy and technology-assisted infants in the home: A comparative study. *Journal of Pediatric Nursing, 14*(3), 164–176.

Strickling, M. V. V. (1993). Home care consumers speak out on quality. *Home Care Nurse, 11*(6), 10–17.

Stullenberger, B., Norris, J., Edgil, A., & Prosser, M. J. (1987). Family adaptation to cystic fibrosis. *Pediatric Nursing, 13,* 29–31.

Taylor, S. G., Renpenning, K. E., Neuman, B. M., & Hart, M. A. (2001). A theory of dependent care: A corollary theory to Orem's Theory of Self-care. *Nursing Science Quarterly, 14*(1), 39–47.

Teague, B., Fleming, J., Wolfe, J., Castle, G., Kiernan, B., Lobo, M., & Riggs, I. (1993). "High-tech" home care for children with chronic health conditions: A pilot study. *Journal of Pediatric Nursing: Nursing Care of Children and Families, 8*(4), 226–231.

Ventura, J. N. (1987). The stresses of parenthood reexamined. *Family Relations, 36,* 26–29.

Wegener, D., & Aday, L. (1989). Home care for ventilator assisted children: Predicting family stress. *Pediatric Nursing, 15,* 371–376.

Chapter 2

Overview of Home Health Care of Children Who Are Technology Dependent

The Office of Technology Assessment's (OTA's) 1987 estimation of children who depend on technology to sustain their lives is shown in Table 2.1. The table presents the categories in which the populations of children were placed and the estimations of the numbers in each

TABLE 2.1   Summary of Office of Technology Assistance Estimates of the Size of the Technology Dependent Child Population, 1987

Defined population	Estimated number of children
Group I:	
Requiring ventilator assistance	680 to 2,000
Group II:	
Requiring parenteral nutrition	350 to 700
Requiring prolonged intravenous drugs	270 to 8,275
Group III:	
Requiring other device-based respiratory or nutritional support	1,000 to 6,000
Rounded subtotal (I + II + III)	2,300 to 17,000
Group IV:	
Requiring apnea monitoring	6,800 to 45,000
Requiring renal dialysis	1,000 to 6,000
Requiring other device-associated nursing	Unknown, perhaps 30,000 or more

of the categories. Because the OTA is no longer operable, it appears, from a review of the literature, that there is no agency in the United States that has prepared similar population estimates. Consequently, it is difficult to ascertain more up-to-date definitive estimates about this population of children on a national basis. Feudtner et al. (2001) indicated that children with complex chronic conditions (CCC) might benefit from pediatric supportive care services, such as home nursing, palliative care, or hospice, especially those children whose conditions are severe enough for death. We do not know, however, the extent of this population or how it is changing over time. The numbers today are likely to be considerably larger for reasons that will be presented later. Many of these medically fragile children are chronically ill and their conditions have an impact on their functioning. Some medically fragile children are technology dependent; cared for in their homes; and are subject to demographic, economic, and attitudinal external factors, according to Rothenberg and Kaplan (1990). Murphy (2001) notes that as medical technology advances, more and more children who are technology dependent are discharged from the hospital early, to be cared for at home. It is evident that the use of technology is maintaining the lives of many children who would have died in the past.

Hobbs, Perrin, and Ireys (1985) estimate that 750,000 children in the United States were living with a variety of chronic health conditions. In 1991 it was estimated that 10 million children in the United States were chronically ill (AACPR, 1998; Stein, 2001). Gortmaker and Sappenfield (1984) note that approximately 10% to 15% of children in the United States have a chronic physical illness or condition. They note that this number translates to about 7.5 million children. Many of these children are technology dependent. The number of children with chronic conditions has increased substantially in recent decades. Consistent technological advances in medical care seem to be a factor in a growing number of children surviving and/or recovering from catastrophic illness, traumatic injuries, and acquired and congenital health conditions. C. E. Smith (1995) indicates several reasons for the growing population of technology-dependent children. They are (1) efficacy and reliability of technology, (2) availability of home care services, (3) cost control measures, and (4) growth in public or consumer demands for life sustaining care.

The effects of care in the home of children who are technology dependent has been placed into three basic categories: physical, psycho-emotional, and psychosocial (Johnson, 1987). Preserving the lives of children by attaching them for long periods of time to technological devices extends not only the lives of human beings but also the definition of being human to include human and machine combinations (Kohrman, 1994). The moral dimension of home care for children who are technology dependent or assisted is another effect that has not provoked as much consideration in the literature as one might expect.

Further demographics reflect that by the year 2020, racial and ethnic minorities, which currently comprise one fourth of the nation's population, will comprise 40% (U.S. H.H.S., 2000). Since minority children tend to have a greater number of chronic health conditions, many may need technology to function adequately.

Home care may be defined as a change in both the location and the focus of care and one that returns care as much as possible to the family and community (Stein & Jessop, 1984). Technological home care is seen as a system of health services delivered by families who manage the care at home of individuals dependent on technology for survival (C. E. Smith, 1995). Care in the home may resemble the hospital where ill persons receive oxygen, dialysis, venous infusions, tube feedings, ventilator care, apnea monitoring, or other technological care. The caregivers are often family members. In the case of the child, the caregiving role in the home may also be assumed by a professional health care worker if the situation or child's needs warrant such. Home care for children who have a significant physical illness, often one that requires technologically sophisticated intervention, may be defined as an attempt to normalize the life of these children in a family and community context and setting, in order to minimize the disruptive impact of the child's condition and to foster the child's maximum growth and development (Stein, 1984).

The concept of home care reflects an aspect of the continuum of progressive patient care. The use of technology in the home to provide health care to individuals is not a new concept. Home ventilator care has been a part of the health care delivery system since the early 1950s, when home care programs were established for polio patients who required ventilation. "High tech" home care is, however, expanding as a result of increasing costs of care. The expectation is that larger numbers of children will be cared for in their homes.

Due to ongoing technological advances in medical care over the past several years, a growing number of children are surviving and/or recovering from catastrophic illness, traumatic injuries, and both acquired and congenital health problems. Many of these children suffer from chronic health conditions and often need highly technical care in both the hospital and the home. They are a diverse group of individuals with a range of conditions who require a broad array of technologies and nursing care.

A general definition of the child who is cared for in the home and requires a mechanical device and substantial daily skilled nursing care to avert death or disability is defined as one who is technology assisted or dependent. Children who have conditions requiring assistance of or dependence on technology for the most part have multisystem conditions, neurological conditions, cancer or hematological disorders, cardiac or respiratory disorders, gastrointestinal disorders, renal disorders, or musculoskeletal disorders.

Based on the literature and the criteria of the National Association of Home Care, the child's medical condition should be stable and the level of support and intervention the child requires should be able to be safely and practically provided in the home before a child who is technology dependent is sent home for care. The family must be motivated and willing to learn the skills and knowledge necessary for the child's care. Family members must also demonstrate proficiency in providing all aspects of the child's care since they will have the primary responsibility. If they are not proficient in providing the care, prepared home health care personnel must be available to provide it. These individuals must be in place before the child goes home. Financial support must be available to fund equipment, supplies, and personnel in the home, and a reliable company must be engaged to provide the necessary equipment and supplies, such as oxygen. The home must be structurally appropriate and it is desirable that community resources such as adequate emotional and respite care are available.

Janz and Burgess (1985) identify components essential to home care quality assurance that seem appropriate to the status of home care today. These structured measures include the education and experience of the staff, standards of care and system review, process measures that consider the plan of care, timelines, and accuracy of the interventions, interdisciplinary involvement, and communication among team members as to the status of the client. Outcome measures that consider goals, functional level, improvement of the client, and client satisfaction are necessary. It is important to emphasize that the family needs support and help from professionals who provide health care services for these children and their families.

The alternative to complex care in the home for many technology-dependent children is to have them remain in the hospital or other health care institutions that can meet their needs. The increase in the delivery of care in the home probably has occurred because of the mandate for cost containment in health care services. Before managed care, home care policy seems to have been shaped to a great extent by Medicaid because patient eligibility and the kinds of services allowed were highly regulated. Home care, more than other health care services, seems to have been influenced by financial reimbursement policies. Managed care may be more of a factor now than Medicaid and the conventional "indemnity" health insurance plans. In the managed care environment, where shorter hospital stays may occur, it is likely that more technology-dependent children with complex care needs may be going home earlier.

Cost containment has thus created a shift toward decreased length of stay in hospitals as well as decreases in services provided and the move to the provision of care in the home. Home care for some chronically ill children who are technology dependent is a reality, whether it is as an alternative or a primary health care delivery source.

Hospitals and health maintenance organizations are purchasing home care agencies. Both public and private agencies are offering home care services. Some hospitals operate their own health care agencies. The concept of home care reflects an aspect of the continuum of progressive patient care. Although many children who are technology dependent are receiving home care, there are those whose needs are complex enough for them to be cared for in the hospital.

An expanding federal health insurance plan for children created an unprecedented opportunity to improve children's health. This plan allocated $20.3 billion for states to use in extended private insurance for children and another $3.6 billion to improve coverage under Medicaid. States must apply for the federal funds and get approval from the U.S. Department of Health and Human Services. The states may need to provide assistance with child care, transportation, culturally appropriate services, better use of information technology to improve access and utilization of service, and other services, identified by knowledgeable persons in the communities to help improve the health care of children.

Exactly how the State Children's Health Insurance Program (SCHIP) has affected or will affect home care of technology-dependent children is not entirely clear. The purpose of SCHIP was to make health insurance available to uninsured children of low-wage working families with incomes too high to qualify for Medicaid but too low to afford private health insurance. Some technology-dependent children who are being cared for in the home are benefiting from this program, considering that the first national enrollment statistics released in 1999 indicated a total enrollment of 982,000 (Insuring America's Children, 2000).

The special and often complex needs of technology-dependent children include medical devices, technical expertise necessary to operate the devices, and professionally trained personnel who can deliver care as needed and provide assistance and monitoring of caregivers in providing technical, nursing, and personal care. Support services for the caregivers are also needed. To help these children reach their full potential for functioning in society, their special needs may include educational, psychosocial, and psycho-emotional assistance with activities of daily living, and physical care to help maintain their basic functions. To ensure that their needs are met, an environment and community conducive to their growth and development is essential.

Some studies have shown that the cost of care is less in the home than in the hospital. The issues of cost and outcome benefits have been studied specifically for ventilator-dependent children, and home care costs were found to be 50% to 95% lower than hospital costs (Burr, Guyer, Todres, Abraham, & Chiodo, 1983). Similar statistics have been noted for dying children (Martinson, 1976). However, little is known about the overall "cost" of care to the family.

Alternatives for delivering care that is both humane and of high quality is imperative in light of the health care financing system. In some cases, home care may be the primary source of care and the hospital the alternative. In other cases home care may be the alternative and the hospital or some other setting the primary source of care.

CLASSIFICATION OF CHILDREN
WHO ARE TECHNOLOGY DEPENDENT

In 1987, the Office of Technology Assessment estimated that between 10,000 and 68,000 of the children who receive care in their home need a medical device to compensate for the loss of a vital body function and substantial and ongoing nursing care to avert death or further disability. Four types of technology assisted or dependent children were described.

Group I—Children who are dependent at least part of each day on mechanical ventilators.

Group II—Children requiring prolonged intravenous administration of nutritional substances or drugs.

Group III—Children with daily dependence on other device-based respiratory or nutritional support, including tracheotomy tube care, suctioning, oxygen support or tube feeding.

Group IV—Children with prolonged dependence on other medical devices which compensate for vital body functions who require daily or near daily nursing care or monitoring. These include: (1) infants requiring cardiorespiratory monitors; (2) children requiring renal dialysis as a consequence of chronic kidney failure; (3) infants requiring apnea monitors; and (4) children requiring other medical devices, such as urinary catheters or colostomy bags, as well as substantial nursing care in connection with their disabilities (see Table 2.1 for estimated numbers of children). While it is possible for children under 20 years of age to have acute conditions and to be technology dependent, most of those receiving home care are children who have a long-term chronic disability; require daily use of a medical device to sustain life and require daily, ongoing skilled care or monitoring.

Understanding the aspects of the family care giving role in the home to these children, the effects, potential outcomes of the care on the children and their families, how to manage and assure that quality care is delivered and the role of professionals in this effort are the primary considerations that will be presented throughout the book.

Fleming et al. (1994) report on a study conducted to create a database that would aid in further describing children who are technology dependent and cared for in their home. Specific aims were (1) to identify select demographic characteristics of children who are technology dependent and their families, (2) to define home care of children who are technology dependent in terms of resources, (3) to test select hypotheses regarding the effects of the illness on the children and their families, and (4) to provide the means for these data to be used by others in the development of recommendations for nursing practice relating to the care of these children and their families. A report of the impact on families from this study indicates some differences in the responses of families (Fleming et al., 1994). Some highlights from this study, along with definitive information from many other research studies that aid in substantiating the care of these children and their families, that may be pertinent to the care of these children are provided in the book.

Three basic assumptions about home care of children who are technology dependent are presented in this chapter.

1. Family-centered care is basic.
   a. When a child who is technology dependent is cared for in the home, the lifestyle of the family changes.

      b.   Family dynamics influence adaptation or maladaptation to situations the family experiences.

      c.   The family's need for information from health professionals depends on several factors and is as important for the caregiver.

      d.   Families are affected in varying ways and need support to cope with the stress of having a child who is technology dependent.

2.   Community integrated services are needed to adequately provide care to this population.

3.   The technological medical device compensates for the loss of use of a body function and helps avert death or further disability.

      a.   Many of the children who are technology dependent and cared for at home are chronically ill.

      b.   The children may have a wide array of diagnoses that affect their systems (respiratory, cardiac, urinary, gastrointestinal, musculoskeletal, etc.)

FAMILY-CENTERED CARE

Caring for a child who is technology dependent in his/her home is basically family-centered. Family-centered care acknowledges the fact that most children live in families and that the family is critical in molding their lives. The health team—nurses, doctors, social workers, and therapists—must always be cognizant of the role the family assumes as caregiver of the child who is being cared for in the home. The trend toward more home health care focuses even more on family-centered care and further acknowledges the critical role that the family has in molding the lives of these children.

The research on the effects of the family environment on the development of children is extensive. It is well documented that interactions in the family affect the whole range of child's development—social, physical, cognitive, and emotional. The family as a system is seen as organizationally complex, that is, a collection of entities interconnected by a complex network of relationships (Kantor & Lehr, 1975). The family network from a systems perspective is open, adaptive, and information processing. Open means there are both internal and external interchanges that can be redefined, depending on what the focus is in the system at any one time. This author believes that strategies that the family uses are generally rational and purposeful. If different strategies seem appropriate in providing care, then these must be taught so that the caregivers become competent. The essential need for information to the caregivers of technology-dependent children cannot be overstated. There are several studies that indicate parents of hospitalized children who receive information have less anxiety, stress, or distress (Bokinskie, 1992; Stinson & McKeever, 1995).

The psychosocial and economic consequences of advances in medical technology that allow for provision of technology-assisted care in the home are somewhat of a dilemma. The dilemma results from the effort of the family to integrate the ill child into the family and manage care that the child would ordinarily receive in the hospital. Balancing the maintenance of the level of care that would be provided by a doctor or a nurse in the hospital in the home results in major adaptations physically, psychologically, socially, and economically on the part of the family.

Family involvement in the care of the child in the home is essential. To assure quality home health care for children, an alliance between the parent and professional is essential (Kirkhart, 1984). O'Brien and Wegner (2002) note that most children who are technology dependent live with their families at home. They explore the perceptions of parents and home care nurses regarding rearing the child who is technology dependent and found that rearing these children is similar to but different from raising other children. Parental communication and negotiation of child-rearing expectations with home care nurses are essential. Kirk (2001), using a grounded theory methodology, finds that from the parents' perspective, the initial assumption of responsibility for the care of their child was not subject to negotiations with professionals. This study supports other research that found that professionals' expectations of parental involvement in the care of sick children role can act as a barrier to negotiating roles. Nurses, according to Kirk, are seen as ideally placed to play the central role not only in ensuring that role negotiation and discussion actually occurs in practice but also in determining the need for appropriate community support services for families. Effective communication between the parental caregiver and the professional is critical to initiating and maintaining an alliance. It is important for professionals to understand the family from a general perspective. If nurses and other professionals want to improve care to children who are technology dependent and being cared for in their home, a greater awareness of sociocultural factors of family dynamics and contemporary aspects of family life is needed.

Accurate assessments of the family are essential in planning and implementing delivery and evaluating the outcomes of care. Understanding the assets and liabilities of the family, interpersonal relationships, roles of members of the family, the developmental level of the family, and the competency of the family is essential to planning and delivering quality care. The family is the nurturing center of human development and the primary agent in both physical and mental health. The family, if supported adequately, is the best bulwark for good mental health in that ties of affection and intimacy can be and are expected to be established. The family can provide the child and other individual members with personal security acceptance, satisfaction, a sense of purpose, companionship, and limit setting. The family begins the acculturation process that, as the child grows and develops, is promoted by other agencies in society.

The Hill and Hansen (1964) framework of family stress still seems applicable today for nurse educators, researchers, and practitioners to use in their roles with families who provide home care to children who are technology dependent. The distinct but interrelated factors of the framework influence the family's ability to cope with the child's illness. Some modifications have been added to the framework to better reflect home care of technology dependent children.

1. Characteristic of the event
   a. Nature of the pathology and system affected
   b. Type of disability
   c. Prognosis
   d. Potential for rehabilitation
   e. Family's perception of the illness
2. Perceived threat to family relationships, status and goals
   a. Past family roles, relations, and communication patterns
   b. The change in the above roles, relations, and patterns secondary to the illness (both real and perceived).
   c. Decision-making patterns before and after the illness
   d. Individual and family "life goals" and changes in life goals secondary to the illness
   e. Feelings on the part of individual family members about the changes in relationships, status, and goals
3. Resources available to the family
   a. Demographic data: household composition, age, sex, educational background, ethnicity, religion, occupation, income, marital status, housing status, transportation available, insurance policies (insurance available)
   b. Persons: family members, friends, and community groups available to the client and family to provide support
   c. Equipment (medical devices) that functions properly
   d. Respite, education, and other services needed

e. Professional health care workers to provide information, training to family, and care to child as needed
4. Past experience with the same or similar situation
   a. Past crisis experienced by the family
   b. Decision-making patterns during the crisis
   c. Individuals identified by the family as ones who can be counted
      on in time of crisis.

COMMUNITY INTEGRATION

The role of the community in integrating services is an important quality
of care dimension that must be considered. Beck, Hammond-Cordero, and
Poole (1994) discuss several aspects of community services for technology-
dependent children. Among those discussed are public health in home
monitoring, the multidisciplinary team involved in the discharge plan
(which includes community agencies/public health services), and transitional discharge planning models. The authors describe the services of
independent community-based home health agencies and highlight benefits
to families, benefits to community agencies and health professions, and
benefits to payers.

More literature is becoming available on children with AIDS who are
technology dependent. The need for respite care is evident as a community
resource that is needed by these children. There also is mention of the
need for coordinated services. There is, however, not extensive literature
available that delineates the importance of coordinated and/or integrated
services needed for families who care for children who are technology
dependent and cared for in their homes.

It is important to recognize that health care does not occur as an isolated
event in the life of a chronically ill child who is technology dependent.
Health care is not independent of other events and factors that impinge
on the children and their families. The integration of community resources
and effective coordination of them to help families is an important dimension of care. Reports of the evaluation of such services so that others can
benefit are critical as these children are throughout the United States and
other parts of the world.

TECHNOLOGY DEVICES

The use of technological devices basically indicates that the individual
child has lost adequate physical functioning in at least one organ system.

Many of the children who are technology dependent are chronically ill. Some are acutely ill or dying. Chronic illness is defined here as (1) an illness that may be permanent caused by a nonreversible pathological condition and that requires long-term supervision or (2) an acquired condition that may be temporary but has existed for at least three months, for which hospitalization or treatment by a physician has been necessary in the past year. From a chronic illness perspective, children who are classified as technology dependent generally are up to 19 years of age with a chronic condition that requires reliance on technology to enable normal functioning or to survive. Many of these children who are on home care have been receiving care for at least one month at home. Some of the devices that are used include respiratory (e.g., nasal cannulae for oxygen, mechanical ventilators, positive airway pressure devices, tracheotomy tubes), surveillance (e.g., cardiorespiratory [apnea] monitors, pulse oximeters), nutritive assistive (e.g., gastrostomy feeding tubes), intravenous therapy (e.g., parenteral nutrition, medication), renal (e.g., dialysis, catherization), or ostomy (e.g., colostomy) devices.

Children who are dependent on a ventilator with or without a tracheotomy need assistance with ventilation; children on oxygen need assistance with oxygenation. The overall survival of some infants has increased because of the success with ventilators and extracorporeal membrane oxygenation. Children who are on dialysis or who have urinary catheters need assistance with elimination of waste products. Children with catheters need special assistance to maintain body functioning by removing excess mucus or other matter. Some receive their nutrients via gastronomy tubes. Children who need IV therapy may need nutritional supplements or pain medication to minimize their pain or treatment for conditions such as cancer. Other devices to help the child maintain adequate bodily functions, such as apnea monitors, vary in accordance with the child's age, diagnosis, length of illness, and other factors.

Reports and observations about the devices and how they affect the children of parents and members of the family who are involved in caring for these children in the home are important. Often their observations of symptoms are essential in ensuring that the medical clinical team makes appropriate clinical decisions in treating these special needs children. The assumption is that quality care will be provided to children regardless of the setting.

LIMITATIONS

Two major limitations seem evident in the provision of home care to children who are technology dependent. They are the difficulty of determining quality of care and the lack of adequate research.

Quality of Care

A major change in health care in the United States seems to be a shift from a provider-centered system to a consumer-driven model. The concern for mandatory reporting of medical errors that result in serious injury or death and voluntary reporting of lesser mistakes along with the proposed establishment of a Center for Quality Improvement and Patient Safety appear to be evidence of greater emphasis on quality of care. This Center, unfortunately, remains a proposal and has not yet been established. Quality of care is seen as a "limitation" because it may be difficult to ascertain what "high quality of care" means in delivering care under a wide array of conditions to children who are assisted by or dependent on one or more technological devices. In a consumer-oriented environment, there likely will be less tolerance of mediocre service and poor quality as indicated by outcomes. Evidence-based practice is emerging as a means that may help facilitate quality care. The role of the community in supporting culturally relevant care for children who are technology dependent may be another quality of care limitation.

Lack of Adequate Research

The limitation of adequate research on which to base practice is a reality. Few experimental or longitudinal studies appear in the literature on the home care of children who are technology dependent. There are, however, a number of descriptive studies and clinically focused articles reported in the 1980s and 1990s that provide useful information about technology-dependent children and, to some extent, their families. Several of these clinically focused articles and studies are presented in the next chapter, as they may be helpful in considering the concepts of evidence-based practice and best practices in the care of children who are technology dependent and cared for in their homes. C. E. Smith (1995) notes that many of the studies done on technology-dependent clients are descriptive and narrow in focus. They are not conceptually or theoretically based. She notes that the model of transitional care advanced by Brooten et al. (1986, 1988) had guided research in comprehensive or family-centered approaches. She states that nurses need research-generated knowledge about mechanisms by which the devices interact with patient physiological states to produce outcomes. There is a need to understand patient and family responses to machine dependency. Smith (1995) suggests the inclusion of culturally diverse populations and longitudinal studies. Priority studies needed, she notes, are studies on the impact of technology in the home, identifying and treating problems of technology dependency, evaluating the caregiving effectiveness of families, and coordinating services for efficient use and access to resources.

The problems associated with home care of children who are technology dependent are complex. Consequently, it is important that longitudinal, experimental, and quasi-experimental studies be conducted to provide more research evidence for practice as the demographics of the nation change and globalization emerges.

SUMMARY

Children who are technology dependent are characterized or classified by the use of a specific medical device that compensates for loss of body function and who require complex daily care to prevent death or further disability. This growing pediatric population of children with special needs is viewed as medically fragile. Home care is seen as a cost-effective and positive alternative for these children to long-term hospitalization. The indirect financial costs that families incur are not usually included in the calculations. Varricchio (1994) indicates that indirect and human costs, then, are paid out-of-pocket, not reimbursed by insurance, or are related to psychological morbidity. They include transportation, medications, respite services, health of the caregiver, family stability, psychic burden, impact on the development of children, and demands on the "sandwich generation." Home care required for technology-dependent children and their families influences the direct as well as indirect costs to the children who are technology dependent, family caregivers, and the community. Parental participation in the delivery of health care in the home is a reality. Newton (2000) points out that the concept of parent participation in family-centered practice has become a central tenet of pediatric nursing for the twenty-first century. The caregiving role of parents requires that they have knowledge necessary to ensure that their children receive competent care.

The chapters that follow provide information that may be useful to nurses, parent caregivers, and other professionals in the delivery of home care to children who are technology dependent and their families. Educators and researchers may also find worthwhile information that they can use in carrying out their roles in preparing students and conducting culturally relevant studies about the home care of children who are technology dependent and their families. Issues related to the importance of accountability, effectiveness of outcomes, quality of care concerns, and patient rights are being addressed more in the health care industry and represent premises that are likely to be reflected throughout the twenty-first century.

REFERENCES

Agency for Health Care Policy and Research. (June 23, 1998). *AACPR Teams with AAHP Foundation to Improve Chronically Ill.* Press Release. Rockville, MD: U.S. Department of Health and Human Services.

Agency for Health Care Policy and Research. (1998). *Children's health 1996 MEPS chartbook no. 1.* (AHCPR Publication No. 98-008). Rockville, MD: U.S. Department of Health and Human Services.

Beck, L. R., Hammond-Cordero, M., & Poole, J. (1994). Integrated services for children who are medically fragile and technology dependent. *Infant Young Children, 6*(3), 75–83.

Bokinskie, J. C. (1992). Family conferences: A method to diminish/transfer anxiety. *Journal of Neuroscience Nursing, 24,* 129–133.

Bowe, L. R., Razmus, C. L., & Giordano, P. (1999). Preparing parents for their child's transfer from PICU to the pediatric floor. *Applied Nursing Research, 12*(3), 114–120.

Brooten, D., Brown, L. P., Hazard-Munro, B., York, R., Cohen, S. M., Roncoli, M., & Hollingsworth, A. (1988). Early discharge and specialist transitional care. *Image: Journal of Nursing Scholarship, 20,* 64–68.

Brooten, D., Kumar, S., Brown, L. P., Butts, P., Finkler, S. A., Bakewell-Sachs, S., Gibbens, A., & Delivoria-Papadopoulous, M. (1986). A randomized clinical trial of early hospital discharge and home follow-up of very-low-birth-weight infants. *New England Journal of Medicine, 315,* 934–939.

Burr, G., Guyer, G., Todres, L., Abraham, B., & Chiodo, T. (1983). Home care for children on respirators. *The New England Journal of Medicine, 309,* 1319–1323.

Farrell, M. F., & Frost, C. (1992). The most important needs of parents of critically ill children: Parents' perceptions. *Intensive and Critical Care Nursing, 8,* 130–139.

Feudtner, C., Hays, R., Haynes, G., Geyer, J. R., Neff, J. M., & Kaepsell, T. D. (2001). Deaths attributed to pediatric complex chronic conditions: National trends and implications for supportive services. *Pediatrics, 107*(6), 1–5.

Fleming, J. (1992). *Home care of technology dependent children.* Unpublished report. Lexington, KY: University of Kentucky.

Fleming, J., Challela, M., Eland, J., Hornick, R., Johnson, P., Martinson, I., Nativio, D., Nokes, K., Riddle, I., Steele, N., Sudela, K., Thomas, R., Turner, Q., Yoshioka, B., & Young, A. (1994). Impact on the family of children who are technology dependent and cared for in the home. *Pediatric Nursing, 20,* 379–388.

Gortmaker, S. L., & Sappenfield, W. (1984). Chronic childhood disorders: Prevalence and impact. *Pediatric Clinics of North America, 31,* 3–18.

Haffner & Shurman (2001)

Hill, R., & Hansen, D. (1964). Families under stress. In H. T. Christensen (Ed.), *Handbook of marriage and family* (pp. 712–819). Chicago: Rand McNally.

Hobbs, N., & Perrin, J. M. (1985). *Issues in the care of children with chronic illness.* San Francisco: Jossey-Bass.

Hobbs, N., Perrin, J. M., & Ireys, H. T. (1985). *Chronically ill children and their families.* San Francisco: Jossey-Bass.

Humphrey, C. J., & Milone-Nuzzo, P. (1991). *Home care nursing: An orientation to practice.* Norwalk, CT: Appleton Century Crofts.

Insuring America's children—a call for nursing participation. (2000, March–April). *Journal of Professional Nursing, 16*(2), 73.

Janz, K. C., & Burgess, B. (1985). Home health care. *Standford Nurse, 7*(3), 9.

Johnson, D. (1987). Possible long-term effects of high technology on the child and family. *Focus on Critical Care, 14*(4), 43–50.

Kahn, L. (1984). Ventilator-dependent children heading home. *Hospitals, 58,* 54–55.

Kantor, D., & Lehr, W. (1975). *Inside the family.* New York: Harper & Row.

Kiernan, B. (1995). Parents' perceptions of family functioning and parental coping in families of chronically ill children dependent upon home intravenous therapy. Doctoral dissertation, University of Kentucky, Lexington.

Kirk, S. (2001). Negotiating lay and professional roles in the care of children with complex health needs. *Journal of Advanced Nursing, 34*(5), 593–602.

Kirkhart, K. (1984). Encouraging early family involvement in home care for children with serious handicapping conditions. *Association for the Care of Children's Health,* 40.

Kohrman, A. F. (1994). Chimeras and odysseys: Toward understanding the technology-dependent child. *The Hastings Center Report, 24*(5), S4(3).

Martinson, I. (1976). *Home care for the dying child.* New York: Appleton Century Crofts.

Maurano (1994)

McCoy, P. A. (1990). Discharge planning. In P. McCoy & W. L. Votroribek (Eds.), *Pediatric home care: A comprehensive approach* (pp. 3–14). Rockville, MD: Aspen Publishers.

Murphy, G. (2001). The technology dependent child at home: Part 1: In whose best interest. *Pediatric Nursing, 13*(7), 14–18.

Newton, M. S. (2000). Family-centered care: Current realities in parent participation. *Pediatric Nursing, 26*(2), 164–168.

O'Brien, M. E., & Wegner, C. B. (2002). Rearing the child who is technology dependent: Perceptions of parents and home care nurses. *Journal of Special Pediatric Nursing, 7*(1), 7–15.

Office of Technology Assessment. (1987). *Technology dependent children: Hospital care vs. home care: A technical memorandum.* Washington, DC: Congress of the United States.

Punch, L. (1985). Pediatric home care expands as technology is developed. *Modern Health Care, 15,* 152, 154.

Rothenberg, R. B., & Kaplan, J. P. (1990). Chronic disease in the 1990s. *Annual Review of Public Health, 11,* 267–296.

Smith, C. E. (1995). Technology and home care. In J. Fitzpatrick & J. Stevenson (Eds.), *Annual Review of Nursing Research, 138,* 143, 153.

Smith, C. E., Giefer, C. K., & Bieker, L. (1991). Technology dependency: A preliminary model and pilot of home total parental nutrition. *Journal of Community Health Nursing, 8,* 245–254.

Smith, S. J. (1991). Promoting family adaptation to the at-home care of the technology dependent child. *Issues in Comprehensive Pediatric Nursing, 14,* 249–258.

Stein, R. (1984). Home care: A challenging opportunity in home care for children with serious handicapping conditions. *Association for the Care of Children's Health, 2.*

Stein, R. (2001). Challenges in long term health care for children. *Ambulatory Pediatrics, 1*(5), 280–288.

Stein, R., & Jessop, D. J. (1984). Does pediatric home care make a difference for children with chronic illness? Findings from the Pediatric Ambulatory Care Treatment Study. *Pediatrics, 73,* 845–853.

Stinson, J., & McKeever, P. (1995). Mother's information needs related to caring for infants at home following cardiac surgery. *Journal of Pediatric Nursing, 10,* 48–57.

U.S. H.H.S. (Department of Health and Human Services). (2000). A national agenda for minority workforce: Racial/ethnic diversity (2000), National Advisory Council on Nursing Education and Practice. Report to the Secretary of Health and Human Services and Congress. Washington, DC: U.S. Department of Health and Human Services, Health Resources and Services Administration, Bureau of Health Professions, Division of Nursing.

Varricchio, C. (1994). Human and indirect costs of home care. *Nursing Outlook, 42,* 151–157.

Chapter 3

Evidence on Home Health
Care of Children Who Are
Technology Dependent and
Their Families

T he purpose of this chapter is to

- highlight the importance of quality care
- briefly indicate a status of evidence for practice
- present an overview of literature that may aid in helping to provide evidence that will enhance the quality of care of children who are technology dependent and their families
- help practitioners, educators, and researchers to identify gaps that need to be addressed in the provision of care for this growing population group

The research cited in this chapter resulted from computer database searches and the review of articles and chapters that deal with home care of technology-dependent children and their families or caregivers.

Quality of Care

Quality of care is an important issue for consumers, professionals, and public policy makers. The standards used in the past to ensure quality are changing. The movement toward a culture of evidence appears to be an emerging issue in the quality of care. When quality of care is presented in the context of evidence-based practice, it is likely to be seen as high quality care. The challenge of addressing how health care can be better for those who need it without incurring exorbitant cost continues to indicate the relevance of many of the issues and positions taken related to quality.

Patients' safety issues emerged as one of the major concerns in 1999–2000. The Institute of Medicine (IOM) and others urged health care systems to reorient their efforts to reduce errors (Bogner, 1994; Cohen, 1999; Spath, 2000). The *To Err is Human* (1999) report from the IOM had a number of recommendations for health care providers, health care and health related institutions, and public policy makers. An Interagency Coordination Task Force, directed by former President of the United States of America Bill Clinton, evaluated and proposed an action plan of the IOM's recommendations: Quality First: Better Health Care for all Americans (2000). The Task Force forwarded a plan to the President virtually endorsing the recommendations from IOM. President Clinton allocated $20 million in the fiscal year 2001 budget to fund a Center for Public Safety, but it has not yet been established. Federal agencies were directed to initiate the Task Force's recommendations. The context of quality in health care seems to be shifting more toward documenting evidence that indicates high quality of care has been or is being provided.

STATUS OF EVIDENCE-BASED PRACTICE

What is evidence-based practice? Evidence of practice seems to be a means to improve decision-making by identifying sound scientific evidence to inform deliberative processes and to ensure safe and quality care for all who enter the health care system regardless of where the care is given. Gerrish and Clayton (1998) state that evidence-based practice uses research findings derived chiefly from randomized controlled, clinical trials or other experimental designs to evaluate specific interventions. Fawcett, Watson, Newman, Walker, and Fitzpatrick (2001) note that what constitutes evidence depends, in part, on what one regards as the basis of evidence. They maintain that theory is the reason for and the value of evidence. Theory and evidence, they indicate, are inextricably linked. Although controversial, they further state that evidence must extend beyond the emphasis of empirical research and randomized clinical trials. Stetler et al. (1998) note that evidence-based nursing stresses the use of research findings and, as appropriate, quality improvement data, other operational and evaluation data, and the consensus of recognized experts to substantiate practice. According to Goode and Piedalue (1999), evidence-based clinical practice involves the synthesis of knowledge from research; retrospective or concurrent chart review; quality improvement and risk data; international, national, and local standards; infection control data; pathophysiological data; cost-effectiveness analysis; benchmarking data; patient preferences; and clinical expertise. Jennings and Loan (2001), in addressing misconceptions among nurses about evidence-based practice, indicate that nurses have voiced strong agreement that evidence-based practice is an important vehicle to improve decisions about the use of limited health care resources for the purpose of maximizing quality care while curbing costs.

There are potent reasons for evidence-based practice. Some of the reasons follow:

1. A decrease in variability across clinician and practice sites. This does not relieve the practitioner of individualizing care based on the specific individual or family for whom care is being provided. Standardized care for specific nursing diagnosis are designed to improve the health and well-being of the individuals for whom care is being provided.
2. A decrease in cost may occur if payers are clear about what the care consists of. Thus, care that is based on evidence-based research findings may affect managed care, as they can make proper assessments of the care.
3. It may help provide a more knowledgeable consumer and delineate more clearly to payers what care has been provided.
4. Providers, patients, and their families may have greater assurance that care is safe, efficient, effective, and reasonably priced.

EVIDENCE-BASED PRACTICE FOR CHILDREN—GENERAL

As noted in Chapter 2, medical advances have resulted in the emergence of a group of children cared for in their homes with chronic health conditions and acute illnesses who are dependent upon technology for their survival. Some terminally ill children who are technology dependent are provided palliative care in their homes. Many of these children's parents and/or guardians are their caregivers in their homes.

Identifying outcomes that are sensitive to multidisciplinary practice is essential to ascertain practices for children who are technology dependent and cared for in their homes. Many of those practices, which are clinically relevant for this targeted population and which are evidence-based, are presented in this chapter.

Accountability on the part of health professionals and parental caregivers of this group of children is a critical factor in establishing practice based on evidence. The goal is for evidence-based practice to help professionals make more effective decisions in providing quality of life symptom management, appropriate health promotion behaviors, and safe care.

Children discharged from hospitals who are technology dependent often require complex home care. To ensure that quality care will be provided, a number of tasks are necessary. Professionals must work with the home caregivers in planning, developing, teaching, and evaluating the care provided to ensure that the outcomes are effective. Outcomes essentially describe what responses should be expected as a result of care and/or treatment.

The systematic review is one of the ways used to establish evidence-based practice. A systematic review is a scientific investigation. One approach is to take the results from several research studies and synthesize them using an approach that limits bias and error. A caution about using systematic review is that it cannot be relied upon solely. Not all outcomes that may be relevant are measured in many studies. Still, systematic reviews are an important tool that can be used to help make practice decisions, particularly as the emphasis on scientific evidence increases and is tied to quality of care.

From a nursing care perspective, quality care would reflect attention to the full range of human experience and responses to health and illness. Integration of objective information and the knowledge gained from the child who is technology dependent and the child's family are the guiding factors in applying scientific knowledge to the process of providing quality care.

The complexity of care of children who are technology dependent and cared for in the home covers a number of factors relevant to the assessment and delivery of nursing care. Among the factors are the diagnosis of the child, age of the child, and family dynamics in the context of support and services. Outcome statements specify the outcomes of supports and services. It is essential to identify outcomes that are sensitive to nursing practice as well as interdisciplinary practices. Issues with such outcomes are the availability of valid and reliable data and linking the data set to the continuum of home care. Outcomes in terms of the management of symptoms, level of functioning, child and family education and information, patient/client satisfaction, and other aspects of nursing care are important to address.

Recognition of the importance of the family and other professionals in outcomes is essential, as patients are not cared for in isolation. The family may influence the outcome in one context while nursing or a professional from another discipline may influence the outcome in another context. Because care of children who are technology dependent is complex, outcomes may be influenced by nursing, the family, and other disciplines. Consequently, when evidence on which to base practice is provided, the strength of the linkages between nursing care and patient outcomes may not be as strong or as clear. An interdisciplinary team approach, of which nursing functions as one of the disciplines in delivering care to these children and their families, is likely to be the focus.

Because children who are technology dependent and being cared for in the home make up a diverse group, the evidence provided in this chapter is limited. Studies are limited not only in terms of the populations studied but also from the perspective of understanding the children and their families. However, the evidence presented in this chapter may provide objective, potentially significant information that will be useful and influence decision-making by families, professionals, and policy makers.

Most of the evidence from research about families and children who are technology dependent and cared for in the home is based on single descriptive studies. The expectation that comprehensive or generalizable knowledge will result from such studies is perhaps not as realistic or convincing as it would be if clinical trials, intervention, and replicated descriptive theory-based and longitudinal studies were done. It is not expected that single descriptive studies would provide definitive explanations of the phenomenon under study. However, some general explanations may be possible about the findings. If an effect is significant, it is an important dimension of a study. This is relevant not only from the perspective of statistically significant tests but also of the statistical power, of which sample size would be a major determinant.

The importance of applying knowledge to practice, education, and the conduct of intervention studies is critical in enhancing the quality of care. The changing health care environment necessitates that evidence serves as the basis for actions in the discovery of new knowledge, transmission of that knowledge, and in practice. The overall effectiveness of health care to this vulnerable population group of children and their families is likely to be enhanced if care is based on evidence. The effectiveness of care, access to resources needed, and satisfaction with care are dimensions of quality to consider with these children (see Figure 3.1).

CLINICAL AND RESEARCH EVIDENCE

There are a number of relevant clinically based articles in the literature that are pertinent to understanding children who are technology dependent

Ardine, C. (1980)	Home care for young children with long-term tracheotomies
Burr, B., Guyer, B., Todres, I., et al. (1983)	Home care for children on respirators
Willis, J. (1983)	Concerns and needs of mothers providing home care for children with tracheotomies
Kettrick, R., Freedman, S., Hornell, D. (1984)	Innovative approaches to facilitating care at home
Moriartz, C., & Wright, R. (1984)	Home oxygen for children
Kopaoz, M., Moriartz, C., & Wright, R. (1985)	Multidisciplinary approach for a patient on home ventilator
Steele, N., & Harrison, B. (1986)	Discharge preparation for technology-assisted children
Aday, L., Aitken, M., & Wegener, D. (1988)	Results of a national evaluation of programs for ventilator-assisted children
Scharer, K., & Dixon, D. M. (1989)	Parents with a ventilator-dependent child
Wegener, D., & Aday, L. (1989)	Home care of ventilator-assisted children
Quint, R. D., Chesterman, E., Crain, L. S., et al. (1990)	Home care for ventilator-dependent children; psychosocial impact on the family
Smith, S. B. (1991)	Promoting family adaptation to at home care of the technology-dependent child
Newacheck, P. W., & Taylor, W. R. (1992)	Chronic illness: prevalence, severity and impact
Abrahamsen, T. G., Sandersen, H., & Bustnes, A. (1996)	Home therapy with subcutaneous immoglobulin infusions in children
Cuttell, Cartland, Angles, & Watson (1996)	Evaluation of a home renal nursing service
Goldman, A (1996)	Home care of the dying child
Haung, F. C., Chang, M. H., & Chen, C. C. (1996)	Home parenteral nutrition in children
Kelly, P., Evans, P., Jordan, A., & Orem, V. (1996)	Care at home for children with cancer
Panitch, H. B., Downes, J. J., Kennedy, J. S., et al. (1996)	Guidelines for home care of children with chronic respiratory insufficiency
Riveria, Stoner, Groothias (1996)	Parental reactions and coping mechanisms
Augenstein, Ward, & Nelson (1997)	Spondyloepiphyseal dysplasia with ventilator dependence
Clayton, M. (1997)	Traction at home

FIGURE 3.1   Select articles about technology-based clinical care and policy.

Holden, C., Sexton, E., & Paul, L. (1997)	Enteral nutrition for children
Megan, K. (1997)	Kids living with AIDS
Noyes, T., Stebbens, V., Sabhan, A., Samuels, M., & Southhall, D. (1997)	Home monitoring of infants
Pilling, M., & Walley, T. (1997)	Parental antibiotics at home in cystic fibrosis
Ribby, K. T., & Cox, K. R. (1997)	Pediatric end-stage renal disease teaching protocol
Petit-de-Mange, E. (1998)	Pediatric considerations in home care
Ledlie, J. W. (1999)	Caregivers to children who have perinatally acquired HIV disease
Hammer, J. (2000)	Home ventilation in children: indications and practical aspects
Hoffner, J. C., & Schenman, S. T. (2001)	The technology-dependent child
Sasaki, M., et al. (2001)	Mechanical ventilation care in severe childhood neurological disorders
Candusso, M., et al. (2002)	Outcome and quality of life in paediatric home parenteral nutrition
Laskey, A., et al. (2002)	Venous air embolism during home infusion

FIGURE 3.1   *(continued)*

and cared for in the home and their families. The importance of knowledge about the child's treatment and the direct or indirect affect on the family emerge in some form in several articles about technology-based clinical care and policy.

Quality of Life

Some research studies provide information about home care, the family, and quality of life. Educators, researchers, and those providing care to children who are technology dependent may find these studies worthwhile (Baumgardner & Burtea, 1998; Colomb, 2000; Feetham, 1984; Goldman, 1996; Holden, 2001; Martin, 1988; Lumeng, Warschausky, Nelson, & Augenstein, 2001; McCubbin, 1989; McCubbin & McCubbin, 1987; Sexton & Holden, 1996; Van Kesteren, Velhuis, & Van-Leyden, 2001).

Standardized questionnaire tools were used by Baldwin, Meyers, and Oppenheimer (1996) to obtain patient data from the perspective of the patient and others providing direct patient care. The purpose of the study was to investigate if home care was a realistic alternative to continued hospitalization of ventilator-dependent adult and pediatric patients. Respondents were asked to measure perceptions of quality of life and quality of care at home versus at the hospital in regard to health status, life satisfaction, emotional well-being, caregiver ability, and professional care and services. Quality of care at home was found to be similar to hospital care. Quality of life was judged to be better at home.

Storytelling assisted families in dealing with the uncertainty of their children's lives, according to Lehna (1999), who examined the statements of mothers obtained as part of a larger study that examined parent care actions for children in home hospice care. Four themes were identified: (1) this pregnancy was not normal; (2) we chose to give birth to our child; (3) my child requires special care; and (4) are you qualified to care for my child? The author concludes that the mother's storytelling assisted the families in dealing with the daily uncertainty of their children's lives. The implications for nursing practice were that health care professionals can support families by listening to their stories and that storytelling is important to families.

There are advantages and disadvantages of a terminal care at home program. The quality of life of the children is thought to be influenced by their happiness at being at home. Some parents may not feel they receive enough information, supervision, support, and preparation for the death of the child.

Quality of life in technology-dependent children and their families was explored by Baumgardner (1999). He found that parents expressed some concerns. Health care professionals do not discuss quality of life issues and the long-term outlook with parents. Families complained that their religious beliefs were ignored when decisions about life support were made, and they were not included in discussions about discontinuing support. Home nursing did increase time available for family activities and optimized the child's medical care, often avoiding hospitalization. Quality of life was defined in terms of physical comfort, institutional status, adequate services, and family/community interaction. Baumgardner's work on quality of life of technology-dependent children and their families notes both positive and negative aspects for families. Home care nursing was highly valued. Growth of individuals in the family was a positive quality of life aspect. Negative effects on the family included physical and mental anguish, inhibitions of normal family functions, and isolation. One of the conclusions drawn is that parents need respite care and advocacy from their health care team.

From 1985 to 1992, a pilot project to investigate home care as a realistic alternative to continued hospital care of adult and pediatric long-term ventilator-dependent patients was carried out at Kaiser Permanente. Using a standardized questionnaire, respondents were asked to measure perceptions of quality of life and quality of care at home versus at the hospital in regard to health status, life satisfaction, emotional well-being, caregiver ability, and professional and personal services. Quality of life was judged to be better at home (Baldwin et al., 1996). The quality of life for children who are technology dependent and cared for in their homes depends to a great extent on the family caregivers and the professional persons who work with them to assure that the care they provide to these children is effective. Lindeman (1992) notes that longitudinal evaluations of caregiver effectiveness are limited. From the literature available today, Lindeman's observation is still pertinent.

Smith (1996) extensively reviewed quality of life home care technologies for both adults and children. Covered are quality of life on nutrition support, ventilation, dialysis, and infusion; family caregiving with specific home care techniques; patient education; cost of caregiving; and future directions of research. The perspective of responses to technology dependence and the challenges that families face in caregiving, becoming educated in technological areas historically used as indicators of quality, patient functional status, illness parameters, longevity, and patient and family members' perceptions of well-being are considered. In her conclusion, she notes that more sensitive evaluations of social isolation, family dysfunction, and long-term impacts of home care are needed, adding that evaluations of the mainstreaming of technology-dependent children into schools and longitudinal studies on caregivers' career disruptions and employment hindrances are also needed. Haddad (1992) and Hoffart (1989) declare that studies addressing home care, ethical, patient, and caregiver education, and quality of life issues should be a part of all future studies. Hegyvary (1983) declares that these issues should be discussed in nursing curricula.

Stress, Coping, Resources, and Support

Sabbeth and Leventhal (1984) found that in 83% of the 34 studies they reviewed on the effect of family adjustment to chronic childhood illness, marital distress was evident. Murphy (1991) provides a perspective on stress and coping of the medically complex child in a study of families as they make their transition from the hospital to home. Kiernan (1995) explores the relationship between family functioning and parental coping in families with chronically ill children who were dependent on home intravenous therapy of nutritional substance and of drug therapy. She found in her cross-sectional study of 97 parents recruited nationally that predictors of the various dimensions of parental coping included age, income, marital status, and family functioning. The ability to function was predicted by coping behaviors and the severity of the child's condition. She concludes that the findings demonstrate that the clinical assessment of the factors may be useful in providing optimal ongoing care and support services to these families. She provides an extensive review of literature on the home care of families with children who are dependent on intravenous therapy. She found that intimate and peer support are significant predictors of family functioning, while marital status significantly predicts intimate and peer support. The notion of positive relationships is connected to the health of the families. Kiernan indicates that the results of her study suggest that parental coping and family functioning provide support for parents' abilities to manage specific technologies in the home. Further research to validate some of the findings in the study is suggested. Family life and parental coping, it appears from her study, are important in the care of IV-dependent children who are receiving care in their home.

Several authors (McCaleb & Luther, 1996; Reed, 1991) describe the coping responses used by parents with technology-assisted or -dependent children and examine the effects that strain and coping responses have on parents' health systems and health promoting behaviors. Family stress theory served as the theoretical framework for the analysis and discussion of parents' responses. Forty mothers and 40 fathers, mean age of 33.9 years, from three states participated in this study. The mean age of the technology-dependent children in this study was 4 years (Smith, Giefer, & Bicker, 1991).

Murphy (1991) notes in a study of stress and coping in the home care of the ventilator-dependent child that the processes must include all members of the family; that while the issues of denial, anger, depression, chronic sorrow, and loss of freedom are not significantly different from those that other families experience, there is an intensity that is different because of the presence of caregivers; and there is a lack of emphasis on vocational and independent living and an intense focus on the medical condition.

Kirk (1998) provides an overview of the literature that examines the experiences of families caring for a technology-dependent child in the home. Thyen, Kuhlthau, and Perrin (1999) examine the way that children with chronic conditions cared for at home and assisted by technology affects maternal employment and child care; the social and clinical factors associated with the decision of a mother to quit employment to care for a child at home; and the way in which care at home and the decision of a mother to quit a job affects maternal mental health. The 6-month post-discharge status of 70 mothers of children assisted by technology was compared with the 6-month post-discharge status of 58 mothers of children matched for age and gender hospitalized for acute illness. Among the results is that the availability of child care had an independent effect on the mothers' decision to quit a job, whereas the severity of the child's condition did not. Child care hours were significantly lower in study group families and were provided mostly by relatives, compared with daycare facilities and regular babysitters in comparison families. Family income was significantly lower in families with a technology-assisted child. Families in the study group had 20 times higher uncompensated health care costs than did the comparison group. Mothers caring for a child assisted by technology reported less good mental health than did the comparison group mothers, and employment seems to mediate this relationship. It was concluded that caring for a child assisted by technology seems to create barriers to maternal employment, diminishing family resources at a time when financial needs actually increase. Lack of family support and child care services increase the likelihood that mothers of children assisted by technology will stay out of the workforce.

Social support of families with special needs children reflects that social support of families is of critical importance (Cassel, 1974; Cobb, 1976; Sabbeth & Leventhal, 1984). Knoll (1992), in an examination of experiences of families, helps define services needed by families who care for children in their homes.

A study by Miles, Holditch-Davis, Burchinal, and Nelson (1999) of mothers with medically fragile infants found that maternal depressive symptoms and developmental impact rating were moderately but negatively correlated at 6 and 16 months. This indicates that higher depressive symptoms are related to more negative developmental impact ratings.

A study of the impact of caregiving on the family of 48 mothers and fathers caring for a medically fragile child at home reveals that factors contributing to a positive parent-professional relationship are professional competence, genuine caring for the child, and respectful, supportive collaboration with the family (Patterson, Jernell, Leonard, & Titus, 1994).

Stephenson (1999) studied 172 families (healthy $N = 87$; technology-assisted $N = 85$). Families completed several instruments. Significant differences between families with healthy and technology-assisted infants were found. Families with technology-assisted infants experience more stressors/ strains and lower levels of well-being than families with healthy infants. Coping, however, for both groups was high. There was no significant difference between the two groups with regard to family coping.

Home Care Technologies

Family adaptation or maladaptation to illness has been addressed by a number of authors (Anderson, 1990; Kiernan, 1995) and is relevant to the evidence-based practice of home health care of technology-dependent children. Miyasaka, Suzuki, Sakai, and Kondo (1997) conducted a prospective study comparing the preceding 6 months and following 6 months of implementation of a videophone system on seven pediatric home respiratory patients and three patients being introduced to home ventilator care. They found large reductions in the number of house calls from physicians, unscheduled hospital visits by patients, and hospital admission days. The investigators conclude that using a special videophone system can now be considered a practical and effective tool to recruit specialist resources into home care and to improve the quality of pediatric home ventilatory service. Smith (1995) has done a creditable job of delineating research conducted on home care technologies. She specifically covers studies on ventilator-dependent children, apnea-monitored infants, and children. She notes that parents of ventilator-dependent children want more timely information about their children's growth, emotional development, schooling, and communication needs. A major limitation of studies on home ventilation, according to Smith (1995), is that outcomes have been defined from a health care (third-party) payer's perspective, emphasizing cost control. She notes that, overall, researchers conclude that family members with a wide range of age, education, and income adequately managed home technology for the ventilated patient.

A number of studies on apnea-monitored infants and children are reviewed by Smith (1995). Her reviews provide information about what mothers experience in caring for their children. She identifies problems that parents report and concerns they have in caring for a child on a monitor. Weakness of the research on apnea-monitored infants and children, according to Smith, is the lack of organizing conceptual frameworks, few prospective longitudinal studies, and dependence on telephone follow-up surveys. Smith's reviews of research on other home care technologies mention some studies that include children. The conclusion and recommendation for research are insightful.

Abrahamsen, Sandersen, and Bustnes (1996) describe their experience with a subcutaneous infusion home therapy program that their institution ran for 6 years. Their evaluation of the subcutaneous therapy of eight patients with immunodeficiency was done by chart review and a questionnaire answered by all of the families. The results reveal that the children were given a total of 1,100 infusions. They started at the age of 2 to 8 (mean = 4.5) years and received infusions for 1.5 to 6 (mean = 3) years. No serious infections occurred. Short-lasting, local side effects such as swelling and redness were frequently reported, but pain or systemic adverse reactions during or after infusions were never encountered. They conclude that home therapy with subcutaneous immunoglobulin infusions in children with congenital immunodeficiencies is a feasible and safe treatment alternative.

Huang, Chang, and Chen (1996) report that home parenteral nutrition (HPN)—a method of feeding pediatric patients with congenital or acquired short bowel syndrome, Crohns' disease, chronic intractable diarrhea, chronic idiopathic intestinal pseudo-obstruction, or Hirschsprung's disease—is a relatively safe feeding method for patients who would otherwise remain hospitalized for prolonged periods on parenteral nutrition for permanent or prolonged intestinal failure. They found that of nine children on home parenteral nutrition, two died, three were moved to oral feedings, and four were continued on HPN. Readmission to the hospital for those patients receiving HPN was reported as acceptably rare.

Twenty-five home parenteral nutrition patients, ages 4 months to more than 13 years, participated in a study in Poland (Ksiazyk et al., 1999), where widespread use of home parenteral nutrition is an obstacle because of lack of interest of commercial companies in delivering feedings to patients. The hospital stays were significantly shorter. There was significant improvement in the weight of the children during therapy, and the costs were 1.6 to 3 times lower than those recorded in other studies. It was concluded that HPN for children with nutrients mixed by caregivers in the home setting is a safe, appropriate method of treatment that can be used in countries where HPN solutions are not manufactured or where commercial HPN is not economically feasible.

A national survey of all children identified on HPN in Sweden revealed that linear growth was normal in nine children, that all of the school-age children attended classes at age-relevant levels, and that families appeared to have adapted and adjusted well (Carlson, Hakansson, Rubensson, & Finkel, 1997).

Starandvik, Hjelte, Malmborg, and Widen (1992) report that 31 patients with cystic fibrosis between the ages of 4 and 7 with *pseudomonas aeruginosa* who were treated with home intravenous antibiotics preferred this type of treatment to hospitalization. Apart from psychosocial advantages, the economical savings were substantial. The home IV antibiotic treatment was safe and effective. Reed (1991) found that children with cystic fibrosis in families who were not coping well in the home tended to be hospitalized more than those of families that were coping well. A conclusion drawn was that it is vital that nurses be able to differentiate between a family having difficulty coping and one that is coping well.

Radford, Thorne, and Bassingthwaighte (1997) interviewed nurses who were experts in the care of children with gastrostomy devices and their families. A secondary analysis of the themes was done from the interviews. Insights of the experts reflect strategies and approaches on the nursing role in caring for children in their home who have gastrostomies. The importance of providing families with clinical practice knowledge, which will help families provide care to these children, is indicated.

Coffman (1997) conducted a phenomenological study to explore the experiences of nurses working with families of children who were technology dependent in their home. A theme emerging from the data of this study is the nurse as a stranger advocating for the child and family. Other themes include collaboration and occupational demands. Manns (2000) explores the long-term influences on mothers' lives who had the experience of caring for a child who has bronchopulmonary dysplasia and is on home oxygen. Her report, from a larger evidence-based qualitative research project, gives voice to 16 mothers who were studied. With the children being out of the hospital for at least a year, the study was specific in providing a long-term perspective.

Thorne, Radford, and Armstrong (1997) document findings from a longitudinal study of how families cope with the caring for a child with a long-term gastrostomy. Revelations about the social, psychological, and technical implications of the gastrostomy are noted both for the children and their families. A comprehensive orientation of how nurses can better support family caregivers coping is provided.

Strauss, Eyman, and Grossman (1996) assess the predictors of mortality in severely disabled children with mental retardation. They compared risk-adjusted mortality rates of those living in institutions with rates of those living in community and found reduced mobility and the use of tube feedings were associated with an increase in mortality risk. Those living in home residence and community care facilities had an estimated 25%

higher risk-adjusted odds on mortality than those in institutions and health facilities. They conclude that a consequence of the current trend toward deinstitutionalization may be an increased mortality rate in children with severe developmental disability.

Colomb (2000) assessed the incident and etiology of central venous catheter-related (CVC) infections in 47 children on home parenteral nutrition. From their findings, they concluded that early CVC infections after home parenteral nutrition onset appear to predict a bad prognosis. Campo et al. (2001) report findings from a retrospective review of patient intravenous antibiotic therapy of children and adults receiving home parental nutrition. They suggest that even in the presence of catheter-related bloodstream infections, if the patient's general condition is good, antibiotic treatment can be safely administered at home.

CONCLUSION

Studies reported have primarily been descriptive studies. The home care of children who are technology dependent is a worldwide issue. Colomb, Goulet, and Ricour (1998) note that the prevalence of home enteral and parenteral programs is rising rapidly all over the world. The status of research studies on children who are technology dependent and cared for at home in the United States and abroad seem to be similar in that most of the studies are also primarily descriptive. Examples of studies from Taiwan, Japan, Sweden, New Zealand, United Kingdom, Poland, and Switzerland are cited here as examples (Campbell, 1998; Carlson et al., 1997; Hammer, 2000; Hooker & Kohler, 1999; Huang et al., 1996; Kamm, Burger, Rimensberger, Knoblauch, & Hammer, 2001; Ksiazyk et al., 1999; Simon et al., 2000; Sakakihara, Yamanaka, Kajk, & Kamoshita, 1998). The study of technology-dependent children and their families is not as extensive as it probably should be, and although the research is primarily descriptive, it is important that it be shared, used, and built upon. Based on the work of Fleming et al. (1994), the review of research on home care technologies by Smith (1995), the caregiving and quality of life in technology home care (Smith, 1999), and the work of many others, more extensive research is still needed to address the complexities and outcomes both positive and negative that affect children and their families. More conceptual and theory-based studies, comparative studies, and longitudinal studies that include culturally diverse populations in society are needed.

Means to determine quality of care in a valid and reliable manner are suspect if we are not certain of our knowledge base. Evidence from some clinically based articles and research provides the means not only to address individual clients but also in some instances to provide assessment tools that will help clinicians obtain data and plan care so that outcomes can be evaluated for their effectiveness. Social and psychological factors emerge prominently as areas in which families need support if they are to carry out the role of caregivers in the home. Nurses are a critical group of professionals who can provide the support families need because of their specialized skills.

As this chapter has indicated, home care with safe equipment, knowledgeable parents, and the support of health care providers is an acceptable option for a wide range of children and youth who are technology dependent. Planning before discharge, along with recognition that health status may change and that families and their children are unique, must be considered in the provision of home care. One consequence of the current trend toward deinstitutionalization may be an increased mortality rate in children with severe developmental disability. Most studies that consider hospital versus home issues reflect that quality and safe care can be provided in the home with adequate support.

There is not explicit evidence that many studies have been replicated or that the subjects studied represent a wide array of cultural or ethnic children and families. C. E. Smith (1999) replicated a study on caregiving effectiveness. There is evidence to support the unique needs of families and their children who are technology dependent and receiving care in their homes.

Most of the children studied were chronically ill and their families were affected in varying ways. Stress on marital relations, deprivation of leisure time, a sense of permanent fatigue, and isolation from parents and siblings are evident in many of these families. Families may experience financial difficulties. The findings of Fleming (2000) about the outcomes of these children and their families reported in the introductory chapter support Smith's notion that more research on long-term lived experiences and outcomes is needed. Educators, researchers, and practitioners have an opportunity to renew and consider the research presented for its efficacy with families and their children who are technology dependent. Researchers like Brooten et al. (1986) and C. E. Smith (1999) have tested models that can be used in nursing with other disciplines. Caregiving effectiveness with technology-dependent children is a challenge for health professionals. Working together, they can design models based on research and evidence that facilitate high-quality, effective care.

REFERENCES

Abrahamsen, T. G., Sandersen, H., & Bustnes, A. (1996). Home therapy with subcutaneous immunoglobulin infusions in children with congenital immunodeficiencies. *Pediatrics, 98*(6 Pt. 1), 1127–1131.

Aday, L., Aitken, M., & Wegener, D. (1988). *Pediatric home care: Results of a national evaluation program for ventilator assisted children.* Chicago: Pluribus Press.

Alexander, S. R., & Honda, M. (1993). Continuous peritoneal dialysis for children: A decade of worldwide growth and development. *Kidney International, 43*(Supp. 40), 565–574.

Anderson, J. M. (1990). Home care management in chronic illness and self-care movement: An analysis of new technologies and economic processes influencing policy decisions. *ANS, 12*(21), 71–83.

Andrews, M., & Nielson, D. W. (1988). Technology dependent children in the home. *Pediatric Nursing, 14*, 111–118, 151.

Aradrine, C. (1980). Home care for young children with long-term tracheotomies. *American Journal of Maternal/Child Nursing, 5*, 121–125.

Augenstein, K. B., Ward, M. J., & Nelson, V. S. (1997). Spondyloepiphyseal dysphasia congenital with ventilator dependence: Two case reports. *Archives of Physical Medicine and Rehabilitation, 77*(11), 1201–1204.

Baldwin-Meyers, A. S., & Oppenheimer, E. A. (1996). Quality of life and quality of care data from a 7-year pilot project for home ventilator patients. *Journal of Ambulatory Care Management, 19*(1), 46–59.

Baumgardner, D. J. (1999). Families at risk: Quality of life in technology-dependent children and their families. *The Exceptional Parent*, 294–29 &3p79(1).

Baumgardner, D. J., & Burtea, E. D. (1998). Quality of life in technology dependent children receiving home care and their families: A qualitative study. *WMJ Official Publication of the State Medical Society of Wisconsin, 97*(8), 51–55.

Bogner, M. (Ed.). (1994). *Human error in medicine.* Hillsdale, NJ: Erlbaum.

Boland, M. G., & Klug, R. M. (1986). AIDS: The implications for home care. *Maternal-Child Nursing Journal, 11*, 404–411.

Bond, N., Phillips, P., & Rollins, J. (1994). Family-centered care at home for families with children who are technology dependent. *Pediatric Nursing, 20*, 123–130.

Bouchard, K. (1998). Issues in case management: Respite care . . . not issues in case management. *Pediatric Nursing, 24*(3), 260.

Brooten, D., Kumar, S., Brown, L. P., Butts, P., Finkler, S. A., Bakewell-Sachs, S., Gibbens, A., & Delivoria-Papadopoulous, M. (1986). A randomized clinical trial of early hospital discharge and home follow-up of very-low-birth-weight infants. *New England Journal of Medicine, 315*, 934–939.

Burr, D. K. (1985). Impact on the family of a chronically ill child. In N. Hobbs & J. M. Perrin (Eds.), *Issues in the care of children with chronic illnesses* (pp. 24–40). San Francisco: Jossey-Bass.

Burr, B., Guyer, B., Todres, I., Abrahams, B., & Chiado, T. (1983). Home care for children on respirators. *New England Journal of Medicine, 309*, 1319–1323.

Campbell, T. (1998). Caring for the technology dependent child—a case study. *Nursing Praxis in New Zealand, 13*(2), 5–10.

Campo, M., Moreno, J. M., Albinana, S., Valero, M. A., Gomis, P., & Leon-Sanz, M. (2001). Outpatient intravenous antibiotic therapy for catheter infections in patients on home parenteral nutrition. *Nutrition in Clinical Practice, 16*(1), 20–24.

Candusso, M., Faraguna, D., Sperli, D., & Dodaro, N. (2002). Outcome and quality of life in paediatric home parenteral nutrition. *Current Opinion in Clinical Nutrition and Metabolic Care, 5*(3), 309–314.

Carlson, G., Hakansson, A., Rubensson, A., & Finkel, Y. (1997). Home parenteral nutrition. *Pediatric Nursing, 23*(3), 272–274.

Cassel, J. (1974). Psychological processes and stress: Theoretical formulations. *International Journal of Health Services, 4,* 471–482.

Chan, J. S. L., & Filippone, A. M. (1998). High-tech pediatric home care: A collaborative approach. *Caring, 17*(5), 30–36.

Clayton, M. (1997). Traction at home: The Doncaster approach. *Pediatric Nursing, 9*(2), 21–23.

Cobb, S. (1976). Social support as a moderator of life stress. *Psychosomatic Medicine, 38,* 300–314.

Coffman, S. (1997). Home-care nurses as strangers in the family. *Western Journal of Nursing Research, 19*(1), 82–96.

Cohen, M. (Ed.). (1999). *Medication errors.* Washington, DC: American Pharmaceutical Association.

Colomb, V. (2000). Economic aspects of paediatric home parenteral nutrition. *Current Opinion in Clinical Nutrition and Metabolic Care, 3*(3), 237–239.

Colomb, V., Faberio, M., Dabbas, M., Goulet, O., Merekx, J., & Ricour, C. (2002). Central venous catheter-related infections in children on long-term home parenteral nutrition. *Clinical Nutrition, 19*(5), 355–359.

Columb, V., Goulet, O., & Ricour, C. (1998). Home enteral and parenteral nutrition in children. *Bailliere's Clinical Gastroenterology, 12*(4), 877–894.

Copen, C. L., & Dedlow, E. R. (1998). Discharging ventilator-dependent children: A continuing challenge. *Journal of Pediatric Nursing: Nursing Care of Children and Families, 13*(3), 175–184.

Cross, D., Leonard, B. J., Skay, C. L., & Rheinberger, M. M. (1998). Extended hospitalization of medically stable children dependent on technology: A focus on mutable family factors. *Issues in Comprehensive Pediatric Nursing, 21*(2), 63–84.

Cuttell, Cartland, Angles, & Watson. (1996). Evaluation of a home renal nursing service. *Paediatric Nursing, 8*(2), 16–18.

Deming, L. M., & Wolf, J. C. (1997). Case management for ventilator-dependent children. *Journal of Care Management, 3*(5), 15–16, 18, 21.

Fawcett, J., Watson, J., Newman, B., Walker, R., & Fitzpatrick, J. (2001). On nursing theories and evidence. *Journal of Nursing Scholarship, 33*(2), 115–119.

Feetham, S. (1984). Family research: Issues and directions for nursing. In H. H. Werley & J. J. Fitzpatrick (Eds.), *Annual review of nursing research, Vol. V* (pp. 3–26). New York: Springer.

Fleming, J., Challela, M., Eland, J., Hornick, R., Johnson, P., Martinson, I., Nativio, D., Nokes, K., Riddle, I., Steele, N., Sudela, K., Thomas, R., Turner, Q., Yoshioka,

B., & Young, A. (1994). Impact on the family of children who are technology dependent and cared for in the home. *Pediatric Nursing, 20,* 379–388.

Fleming, J., & Barron, M. (2000). Follow-up Study "High Tech" Home Care of Technology Dependent Children with Chronic Health Conditions. Unpublished report. College of Nursing. University of Kentucky, Lexington, KY.

Gerrish, K., & Clayton, J. (1998). Improving clinical effectiveness through and evidenced based approach: Meeting the challenges for nursing in the United Kingdom. *Nursing Administration Quarterly, 22*(4), 55–65.

Goldman, A. (1996). Home care of the dying child. *Journal of Palliative Care, 12*(3), 16–19.

Goode, C. J., & Piedalue, B. (1999). Evidence-based clinical practice. *Journal of Nursing Administration, 29*(6), 15–21.

Haddad, A. M. (1992). Ethical problems in home care. *Journal of Nursing Administration,* 22(3), 46–51.

Haffner, J. C., & Schurman, S. J. (2001). The technology dependent child. *Pediatric Clinics of North America, 48*(3), 751–764.

Hammer, J. (2000). Home mechanical ventilation in children: Indications and practical aspects. *Schweizerische Medizinische Wochenschrift, 130*(49), 894–902.

Hazelette, D. (1989). A study of pediatric home ventilator management: Medical, psychosocial and financial aspects. *Journal of Pediatric Nursing, 4*(4), 284–293.

Hegyvary, S. T. (1983). *A vision for nursing education.* New York: National League for Nursing.

Hoffart, N. (1989). Nephrology nursing 1915–1970: A historical study of the integration of technology care. *American Nephrology Nurse's Association Journal, 16,* 169–178.

Holden, C. (2001). Review of home paediatric parenteral nutrition in the UK. *British Journal of Nursing, 10*(12), 782–788.

Holden, C., Sexton, E., & Paul, L. (1997). Enteral nutrition for children. *Nursing Standard, 11*(32), 49–56.

Hooker, L., & Kohler, J. (1999). Safety, efficacy and acceptability of home intravenous therapy administered by parents of pediatric oncology patients. *Medical Pediatric Oncology, 32*(6), 421–426.

Huang, F. C., Chang, M. H., & Chen, C. C. (1996). Home parenteral nutrition in children. *Journal Formos Medical Association, 95*(1), 45–50.

Institute of Medicine. (1999). *To err is human: Building a safer health care system.* Washington, DC: Institute of Medicine.

Jackson, D. F. (1986). Nursing care plan: Home management of children with BPD. *Pediatric Nursing, 12*(5), 342–347.

Jennings, B. M., & Loan, L. (2001). Misconceptions among nurses about evidence based practice. *Journal of Nursing Scholarship, 33*(2), 121–126.

Kamm, M., Burger, R., Rimensberger, P., Knoblauch, A., & Hammer, J. (2001). A survey of children supported by long-term mechanical ventilation in Switzerland. *Swiss Medical Weekly, 131*(19–20), 261–266.

Kelly, P., Evans, M., Jordan, A., & Orem, V. (1996). Developing a new method to record care at home for children with cancer: An example of research and practice collaboration in a regional pediatric oncology unit. *European Journal of Cancer Care,* 5(1), 26–31.

Kettrick, R., Freedman, S., & Hornell, D. (1984). Innovative approaches to facilitating care at home: Association for the care of children's health: Home care for children's health. *Home Care for Children with Serious Handicapping Conditions*, 9–19.

Kiernan, B. (1995). Parents' perception of family functioning and parental coping in families of chronically ill children dependent upon home intravenous therapy. Doctoral dissertation, University of Kentucky, Lexington.

Kirk, S. (1998). Families' experiences of caring at home for a technology dependent child: A review of literature. *Child Care, Health and Development*, 24(2), 101–114.

Knoll, J. (1992). Being a family: The experience of raising a child with a disability or chronic illness [Monograph]. *American Association of Mental Retardation*, 18, 9–56.

Kopaoz, M., & Moriartz-Wright, R. (1984). Multidisciplinary approach for the patient on a home ventilator. *Heart and Lung*, 13, 255–262.

Ksiazyk, K. J., Lyszowska, M., Kierkus, J., Bogucki, K., Ratynska, A., Tondys, B., & Sacha, J. (1999). Home parenteral nutrition in children: The Polish experience. *Journal of Pediatric Gastroenteralogrand Nutrition*, 28(2), 132–136.

Laskey, A., Dyer, C., & Tobias, J. D. (2003). Venous air embolism during home infusion therapy. *Pediatrics*, 109(1), E15.

Ledlie, S. W. (1999). Diagnosis disclosure by family caregivers to children who have perinatally acquired HIV disease: When the time comes. *Nursing Research*, 48(3), 141–149.

Lehna, C. (1999). Storytelling in practice: Part one—mothers' stories. *Journal of Hospice and Palliative Nursing*, 1(1), 21–25.

Lindeman, C. A. (1992). Nursing and technology: Moving into the 21st century. *Caring*, 11(9), 7–10.

Lumeng, J. C., Warschausky, S. A., Nelson, V. S., & Augenstein, K. (2001). The quality of life of ventilator-assisted children. *Pediatric Rehabilitation*, 4(1), 21–27.

Manns, S. V. (2000). Life after SCBU: The long-term effects on mothers at home with a child with bronchopulmonary dysplasia and on home oxygen. *Journal of Neonatal Nursing*, 6(6), 193–196.

Martin, K. (1988). Research in home care. *Nursing Clinics of North America*, 23, 373–385.

McCaleb, A., & Luther, L. S. (1996). Characteristics and coping patterns of families with infants on home apnea monitoring. *Issues in Comprehensive Pediatric Nursing*, 19(2), 81–92.

McCubbin, M. A. (1989). Family stress and family strengths: A comparison of single and two-parent families with handicapped children. *Research in Nursing and Health*, 12, 101–110.

McCubbin, M. A., & McCubbin, H. I. (1987). Family stress theory and assessment. In H. I. McCubbin & A. I. Thompson (Eds.), *Family assessment inventories for research and practice* (pp. 3–32). Madison, WI: University of Wisconsin-Madisonville.

Megan, K. (1997). Kids living with AIDS. *Journal of HIV-AIDS—Prevention and Education for Adolescents and Children*, 1(2), 7–12.

Miles, M. S., Holditch-Davis, D., Burchinal, P., & Nelson, D. (1999). Distress and growth outcomes of mothers of medically fragile infants. *Nursing Research*, 48(3), 129–140.

Miller, V. L., Rice, J. C., DeVoe, M., & Fos, P. J. (1998). The analysis of program and family costs of case management care for technology dependent infants with bronchopulmonary dysphasia. *Journal of Pediatric Nursing*, 13(4), 244–251.

Miyasaka, K., Suzuki, Y., Sakai, H., & Kondo, Y. (1997). Interactive communication in high technology home care: Video phones for pediatric ventilator care. *Pediatrics,* (1), E1.

Murphy, K. (1991). Stress and coping in home care: A study of families. In N. J. Hochstudt & D. Yost (Eds.), *The medically complex child: The transition to home care* (pp. 287–302). New York: Harwood Academic Publishers.

Newacheck, P. W., & Taylor, W. R. (1992). Chronic childhood illness: Prevalence, severity and impact. *American Journal of Public Health, 82,* 364–371.

Noyes, J., Stebbens, V., Sobhan, G., Samuels, M. & Southall, D. (1996). Home monitoring of infants at increased risk of sudden death. *Journal of Clinical Nursing, 5*(5), 297–306.

Panitch, H. B., Downes, J. J., Kennedy, J. S., Kolb, S. M., Parra, M. M., Peacock, J., & Thompson, M. C. (1996). Guidelines for home care of children with chronic respiratory insufficiency. *Pediatric Pulmonol, 21*(1), 52–56.

Patterson, J. H., Jernell, J., Leonard, B. J., & Titus, J. C. (1994). Caring for medically fragile children at home: The parent-professional relationship. *Journal of Pediatric Nursing, 9*(2), 98–106.

Petit-de-Mange, E. A. (1998). Pediatric considerations in home care. *Critical Care Nursing Clinics of North America, 10*(3), 339–346.

Petr, C. G., Murdock, B., & Chapin, R. (1995). Home care for children dependent on medical technology: The family perspective. *Social Work Health Care, 21*(1), 5–22.

Pilling, M., & Walley, T. (1997). Parenteral antibiotics at home in cystic fibrosis: Experiences and attitudes of recipients. *Health and Social Care in the Community, 5*(3), 209–212.

Quality First: Better health care for all Americans: Final report to the President of the United States/The President's Advisory Commission on Consumer Protection and Quality Health Care Industry. (1998). Washington, DC: The Commission. G.P.O. Superintendent of Documents.

Quint, R. D., Chesterman, E., Crain, L. S., Winkleby, M., & Boyce, W. T. (1990). Home care of ventilator dependent children: Psychosocial impact on the family. *American Journal of Diseases of Children, 144*(11), 1238–1241.

Radford, M. J., Thorne, S., & Bassingthwaighte, C. (1997). Long-term gastrostomy in children: Insights from expert nurses. *Issues in Comprehensive Pediatric Nursing, 20*(1), 35–50.

Reed, S. B. (1991). Potential alterations in family process: When a family has a child with cystic fibrosis. *International Disability Study, 13*(4), 146–149.

Ribby, K. J., & Cox, K. R. (1997). Organization and development of a pediatric end-stage renal disease teaching protocol for peritoneal dialysis. *Pediatric Nursing, 23*(4), 393–399.

Rivera, S. J., Stoner, M., & Groothuis, J. (1996). Caring for a chronically ill child at home: Parental reactions and coping mechanisms. *Home Health Care Management and Practice, 8*(4), 56–63.

Sabbeth, B., & Leventhal, J. (1984). Marital adjustment to chronic childhood illness: A critique of literature. *Pediatrics, 93,* 762–767.

Sakakihara, Y., Yamanaka, T., Kajk, M., & Kamoshita, S. (1996). Long-term ventilator-assisted children in Japan: A national survey. *Acta Pediatrica Japonica, 38*(2), 137–142.

Sasaki, M., Sugai, K., Fukomizu, M., Hanaoka, S., & Kaga, M. (2001). Mechanical ventilation care in severe childhood neurological disorder. *Brain and Development*, 23(8), 796–800.

Scharer, K., & Dixon, D. M. (1989). Managing chronic illness: Parents with a ventilator-dependent child. *Journal of Pediatric Nursing*, 4, 236–247.

Sexton, E., Paul, L., & Holden, C. (1996). A pictorial assisted teaching tool for families. *Pediatric Nursing*, 8(5), 24–26.

Shipley, L. (1997). Technology dependent children at home. *Nursing in Critical Care*, 2(5), 235–238.

Simon, A., Fleischhack, G., Hasan, C., Bode, V., Englehart, S., & Kramer, M. H. (2000). Surveillance for nosocomial and central line related infections among pediatric hematology-oncology patients. *Infection Control and Hospital Epidemiology*, 21(9), 592–596.

Sirkia, K., Saarinen, V. M., Ahlgren, B., & Hovi, L. (1997). Terminal care of the child with cancer at home. *ACTA Pediatrics*, 86(10), 1125–1130.

Smith, C. E. (1995). Technology and home care. In J. Fitzpatrick & J. Stevenson (Eds.), *Annual Review of Nursing Research*, 138, 143, 153.

Smith, C. E. (1999). Caregiving effectiveness in families managing complex technology at home: Replication of a model. *Nursing Research*, 48(3), 120–128.

Smith, C. (1996). Caregiving and quality of life in technological home care: Part II. In J. Fitzpatrick, A. Jacox, & J. Norbeck (Eds.), *Annual Review of Nursing Research* (Vol. 14, pp. 95–118). New York: Springer.

Smith, C. E., Giefer, C. K., & Bicker, L. (1991). Technology dependency: A preliminary model and pilot of home total parental nutrition. *Journal of Community Health Nursing*, 8, 245–254.

Smith, S. J. (1991). Promoting family adaptation to the at-home care of the technology dependent child. *Issues in Comprehensive Pediatric Nursing*, 14, 249–258.

Spath, P. (Ed.). (2000). *Error reduction in health care*. San Francisco: Jossey-Bass.

Starandvik, B., Hjelte, L., Malmborg, A. S., & Widen, B. (1992). Home intravenous antibiotic treatment of patients with cystic fibrosis. *Acta Paediatric*, 81(4), 340–344.

Steele, N., & Harrison, B. (1986). Technology assisted children: Assessing discharge preparation. *Journal of Pediatric Nursing*, 1, 150–158.

Stephenson, C. (1999). Well-being of families with healthy and technology assisted infants in the home: A comparative study. *Journal of Pediatric Nursing: Nursing Care of Children and Families*, 14(3), 164–176.

Stetler, C. B., Brunell, M., Givliano, K. K., Morsi, D., Prince, L., & Newell-Stoke, V. (1998). Evidence-based practice and the role of nursing leadership. *Journal of Nursing Administration*, 28(7–8), 45–53.

Strauss, D., Eyman, R. K., & Grossman, H. J. (1996). Predictors of mortality in children with severe mental retardation: The effect of placement. *American Journal of Public Health*, 86(10), 1422–1429.

Thorne, S. E., Radford, M. A., & Armstrong, E. (1997). Long-term gastrostomy in children: Caregiver coping. *Gastroenterology Nursing*, 20(2), 46–53.

Thyen, U., Kuhlthau, K., & Perrin, J. M. (1999). Employment, childcare and mental health of mothers caring for children assisted by technology. *Pediatrics*, 103(6PTI), 1235–1242.

Van Kesteren, R. G., Velhuis, B., & Van-Leyden, L. W. (2001). Psychosocial problems arising from home ventilation. *American Journal of Physical Medicine and Rehabilitation, 80*(6), 439–446.

Wegener, D., & Aday, L. (1989). Home care for ventilator assisted children: Predicting family stress. *Pediatric Nursing, 15,* 371–376.

Wills, J. (1983). Concerns and needs of mothers providing home care for children with tracheotomies. *Maternal Child Nursing Journal, 12*(2), 89–107.

Youngblut, J. M., & Brooten, D. (2000). Moving research into practice: A new partner. *Nursing Outlook, 48*(2), 55–56.

Chapter 4

Description and Results of a Major Study of "High Tech" Home Care for Children with Chronic Health Conditions

This chapter describes the study by Fleming et al. (1993) of 898 technology-dependent children, on which much of this book is based. The purpose of this study was to further describe technology-dependent children and their families by examining various constructs and testing specific hypotheses. Four types of dependencies were the independent variables. Covariants were those that may affect responses but were not controlled by the investigator. These include duration of condition; regions of the country; demographic information such as economic status; cost of care; perception of resources; and type of agency (public/private) from which services were received. Dependent variables were the responses that result in terms of depression and satisfaction. Mediating variables were family stress, impact, social support, and the child's developmental level.

RESEARCH OBJECTIVES

The objective of the study was to create a database that will aid in further describing children who are technology dependent and being cared for in their homes. The specific aims were to

1. Identify selected demographic characteristics of children who are technology dependent and their families
2. Define home care of children who are technology dependent in terms of consumption of resources

3. Test selected hypotheses regarding the effects of the illness of these children on their families. (The hypotheses tested are listed here; see Figure 1 for the conceptual schema for testing the hypotheses)

> *Hypothesis 1:* There will be a difference in the family level of stress in the families of ventilator-dependent (VD) children, children receiving IV therapy, children with daily dependence on specific support devices (SSDs), and children requiring monitoring of vital functions (VFs).
>
> *Hypothesis 2:* There will be a difference in the impact on the family in the families of VD children, children receiving IV, children with daily dependence on SSDs, and children requiring monitoring for VFs.
>
> *Hypothesis 3:* There will be a difference in the adaptive behavior of VD children, children receiving IV therapy, children with daily dependence on SSDs, and children requiring monitoring for VFs.
>
> *Hypothesis 4:* There will be a difference in the social support of the family of VD children, children receiving IV therapy, children with daily dependence on SSDs, and children requiring monitoring of VFs.
>
> *Hypothesis 5:* There will be a difference in the level of parent's depression for VD children, children receiving IV therapy, children with daily dependence on SSDs, and children requiring monitoring for VFs.
>
> *Hypothesis 6:* There will be a difference in the level of satisfaction in VD children, children receiving IV therapy, children with daily dependence on SSDs, and children requiring monitoring for VFs.
>
> *Hypothesis 7:* The type of dependence affects the family stress level, the impact on the family, the child's adaptive behavior level, and the amount of social support, which in turn determines the caregiver's level of depression and level of satisfaction.

4. Provide means for these data to be used by others in the development of recommendations for nursing practice as they related to the care of children who are technology dependent and their families.

Each of the four objectives incorporates several components.

1. To identify the select demographic characteristics of the population of technology dependent children who are cared for in the home and their families

    a. Age/sex/race of children
    b. Family constellation, structure, and dynamics
    c. Etiology of conditions and diagnosis
       1) Permanent
       2) Temporary
       3) Length of condition
       4) Severity of condition
       5) Length of time cared for in the home
    d. Type of dependency using classifications from Office of Technology Assessment (1987)
2. To define this population from perspective of consumption of resources
    a. Units of nursing care regarding types of care given (i.e., suctioning, gastrostomy feeding, intravenous medications, etc.), those who give care (i.e., aide, L.P.N., R.N., etc.), and number and length of visits
    b. Cost of care required and payment sources
    c. Community and other resources
    d. Family supports and coping resources
    e. Public or private agency involvement
3. To determine the effect of the dependency on the family
    a. The impact of care on the family
    b. Social support for the family
    c. Stress on the family (psychological and physiological)
    d. Parent and sibling responses
    e. Adaptive development behavior
4. To integrate this data into a form capable of supporting development of standards for nursing practice, education, and continuing support of nurses providing care for technology-dependent children and their families in the home settings

A technology-dependent/assisted child is defined as "one who needs both a medical device to compensate for the loss of a vital body function and substantial and ongoing nursing care to avert death or further disability" (OTA, 1987, p. 3). The OTA delineated four separate populations, distinguished by their clinical characteristics. These definitions were used in this project. The groups are defined as follows:

Group I: Children dependent at least part of each day on mechanical ventilators

Group II: Children requiring prolonged intravenous administration of nutritional substances or drugs

Group III: Children with daily dependence on other device-based respiratory or nutritional support, including tracheotomy tube care, suctioning, oxygen support, or tube feeding

Group IV: Children with prolonged dependence on other medical devices that compensate for vital body functions who require daily or near daily nursing care. This group includes

- infants requiring apnea (cardiorespiratory) monitors
- children requiring renal dialysis as a consequence of chronic kidney failure
- children requiring other medical devices, such as urinary catheters or colostomy bags, as well as substantial nursing care in connection with their disabilities (OTA, 1987, p. 4).

Dependent variables were the responses that result in either depression and satisfaction. Mediating variables were family stress, impact, social support, and the child's developmental level. Covariants were those that may have affected responses but were not controlled by the investigator. These include duration of condition, regions of the country, demographic information such as economic status, cost of care, perception of resources, and type of agency (public/private) from which services were received.

Study Design and Methods

The study was a descriptive survey. A purposive sample was obtained from families receiving services from both public and private agencies in 13 cities representing geographic census regions of the country. A structured telephone interview was conducted with the primary caregiver (parent or guardian) of the technology-dependent child. Children were between 3 months and 19 years of age and had been technology dependent and being cared for at home for at least 1 month.

In each of the cities, a nurse served as a coinvestigator/liaison consultant for the study. The areas were representative of the regions and subregions identified from the U.S. Census Bureau definitions. Data were obtained through a structured telephone interview conducted by the University of Kentucky Survey Research Center. The parents or primary caregivers of technology-dependent children were the subjects, and each was interviewed. The children represented a mixture of those receiving services from both public and private home health agencies. The children were also representative of all four groups of technology dependency as defined by the OTA (1987).

To avoid bias and logistical problems, a three-stage sampling procedure was used. At Stage I, each liaison consultant listed and briefly described a maximum of 10 home care agencies, equipment vendors, and tertiary care hospitals with pediatric home care units in his or her area that cared for technology-dependent children. Also at Stage I, the university research team selected a subset of these agencies for further sampling; criteria were the number and mix of children that reflected the groups of children defined as technology dependent by the OTA (1987). At Stage II, each liaison consultant worked with those selected agencies in compiling lists of families who were to be sampled and sent letters seeking participation in the study. Hence, consultants were primarily responsible for recruiting agencies, while selected volunteer agencies were responsible for recruiting volunteer caregivers. They avoided problems that would have occurred in attempting to satisfy numerous internal review boards on the issue of protecting patient privacy.

Each selected volunteer agency compiled two lists of names by using the following patient stratification:

Strata A: Children with a prolonged dependence on a medical device that is required to sustain life. Using the OTA manual, this included the following three groups of children:

Group I: Children dependent as least part of the day on mechanical ventilators

Group II: Children requiring prolonged intravenous administration of nutritional substances or drugs

Group III: Children with daily dependence on other device-based respiratory or nutritional support, including tracheotomy tube care, suctioning, oxygen support, or tube feedings

Strata B: Children with a prolonged dependence on other medical devices that compensate for vital body functions who require daily or near daily nursing care. This includes

- Children requiring apnea (cardiorespiratory) monitors
- Children requiring renal dialysis as a consequence of chronic renal failure

- Children requiring devices such as urinary catheters or colostomy bags as well as substantial nursing care in connection with their disabilities

Once these lists were constructed, each selected agency was requested to send information packets describing the purpose of the study (which had been provided to them) to a subset of the caregivers of patients on the lists. The number of names selected from each list was determined by the University of Kentucky research team; a systematic sample was the method for choosing names. The information packet contained a description of the purpose of the study and an addressed postcard. Caregivers, most of whom were parents interested in volunteering for the study, were asked to complete the postcard (name, telephone number, and child's type of dependency) and mail it to the university research team. They were provided information about the study and told how their rights would be protected.

Stage III occurred once the postcards were returned. The final sample, with approximately 40 per strata per region, was made up of those who returned the postcards, indicating their willingness to participate. Each person was called to arrange a time for the interview. An interviewer, trained by team personnel, called at the scheduled time using the structured interview guide, which consisted of demographic information, select published scales, and investigator-developed questions. Permission had been obtained to use the select published scales. A protocol approved by the Human Subjects Review Committee was followed to ensure that subjects' rights were protected. The interview guide was pilot tested before being use in major study.

Measures

Measures obtained in the study follow.

Family Inventory of Life Events (FILE)

This self-report assessment-designed instrument measured family stress by recording normative and nonnormative family demands that the family might have experienced in the past year (McCubbin & Patterson, 1981). The latest adaptation of the inventory (Form C) was used. This form contains nine subscales and includes items that focus on family demands and strains associated with a chronically ill family member. The total index is reliable with a Cronbach alpha of .81. Tests of validity indicated the total inventory score is significantly and inversely correlated with measures of changes in health states, and that this score is correlated significantly with measures of family functioning.

Impact on Family Scale

This scale was designed to measure the effect of a child with a chronic condition in producing change in the family (Stein & Riesman, 1982). Impact was conceptualized as the effects of the child's illness on the family system. Four dimensions were theorized as relevant: economic (changes in the economic status of the family), social (quality and quantity of interactions with others outside the family), familial (quality of interaction within the family unit), and strain (subjective burden experienced by the primary caretaker). The scale is seen as reliable enough to detect a change in the family's lifestyle. The construct validity had been extended, and the analyses of the data of 209 cases suggest that the Impact on Family Scale was tapping the construct it was designed to measure.

Social Support Inventory (SSI)

This scale provides an index of social support that was available and that the caregiver received from various sources as perceived by the caregiver (McCubbin & Thompson, 1987). Reliability was reported at .82 level.

Center for Epidemiological Studies Depression (CES-D) Scale

This 20-item scale assesses depressive symptomology over the previous 7-day period. It attempts to gauge the feelings of the caregiver within the past week. Internal consistency with this scale had been demonstrated at the .85 level or above (Radloff, 1977).

Family APGAR

Caregiver satisfaction is measured with this five-item scale developed by Smilkstein (1978). It was used to obtain information on caregiver's satisfaction. It had been found to have satisfactory internal consistency reliability (alpha = .80), test-retest reliability ($r = .83$), and validity in previous research (Austin & Hubety, 1989).

Child's Development

Parents were asked questions about their children's development. The caregiver was asked if the child's development had been assessed by a health professional and, if so, if there were developmental problems. The caregiver also was asked to evaluate the child's level of functioning compared with other children of the same age. If delays were present, they were also asked to identify the area or domain of the delay.

Demographics

The child's age, gender, race, primary medical diagnosis, and technology dependency were recorded. Also recorded were the caregiver's age; relationship to child; education; marital status; work status; residence; number of children in the family; religious preference; family income; transportation; and resources.

An advisory committee composed of nurses serving as liaisons/consultants to the project and who are involved directly or indirectly in the delivery of home care and parents of children who are technology dependent and receiving home care provided input to the principal investigator about the proposed methodology. A pilot study was conducted to ensure that the data proposed and the approach to be used to obtain information about the development of children would be obtainable. The database was to be used to develop standards for practice, establish professional policy regarding nursing practice, and continue support of nurses providing home care to technology dependent children with chronic conditions and their families. The database may also be useful in planning for continuity of care, interdisciplinary collaboration, curriculum development for nursing programs, and further research. The database may also be used to disseminate information that could provide insight into means of supporting these families. The study was approved by the Institutional Review Board of the University of Kentucky.

FINDINGS

Demographics

The primary caregivers of 848 technology-dependent children were interviewed. The caregivers ranged in age from 17 to 65 years with 49.3% being between 25 and 34 years. Eighty-eight percent of the children were cared for by their mothers, with the other 12% of the caregivers being fathers, foster parents, adoptive parents, or others. Seventy-seven percent of the caregivers were married; 42% were currently working outside of the home and 58% were not.

Fifty-seven percent of the children were males and 43% were females: 10.7% were ventilator dependent, with a mean age of 6.9 years ($SD = 5.4$); 13.8% were IV dependent, with a mean age of 6.7 years ($SD = 5.0$); 50.1% were dependent on devices such as feeding tubes or oxygen support, with a mean age of 4.0 years ($SD = 3.9$); and 25.4% used monitoring devices, with a mean age of 2.1 years ($SD = 3.7$). Their primary medical diagnoses varied (see Table 5.1 in Chapter 5 for overall description of demographics of the 848 participants).

Hypotheses 1

A significant difference was found among the mean profiles of the four dependency groups on the nine subscales of the Family Inventory of Life Events (MANOVA $F = 5.98$ based on 27 and 2,439 degrees of freedom, $p = 0.0001$). To explain this significant difference further, a one-way analysis was used to compare means among the four types of dependency groups for each subscale. Significant differences were found for three subscales— family life change, pregnancy and childbearing strains, and illness and family care strains.

Hypothesis 2

A significant difference was found among the four types of dependencies on the mean profiles for the subscales of the Impact on Family (MANOVA $F = 9.43$ based on 12 and 2223 degrees of freedom, $p = 0.0001$). A one-way ANOVA F test showed that the means vary among the subscales for financial burden, family social impact, and personal strain.

Hypothesis 3

A significant difference was found in the variance of adaptive behavior of children with the type of dependency (Chi Square = 132.8, 3df, $p = 0.001$).

Hypothesis 4

Mean social support was found to not vary significantly among the four types of dependencies.

Hypothesis 5

Mean depression scores did not vary significantly among the four types of dependencies. A significant correlation was found between the family stress score (total score of the nine subscales of the FILE) and the actual depression (CES-D) score ($= .47$, $p < 0.0001$).

Hypothesis 6

Three measures of satisfaction were made, two of which were not found to be significant. The third measure, satisfaction with the quality of the caregiver's life in general, varied significantly among the four types of dependencies (Chi Square $= 31.2$, 3df, $p = 0.0001$).

Hypothesis 7

While the type of dependency affects family stress level, impact on the family, adaptive behavior level of the child, and the amount of social support, once these factors are controlled for by type of dependency, there is basically no effect on the caregiver's level of depression or satisfaction. A logistic regression model was used to predict the log odds of respondents with a CES-D score of 16 or above (indicating signs of depression), a Family APGAR score above the median (indicating satisfaction) reporting a great deal of satisfaction with having enough finances to provide an adequate level of care for their child. The results of this analysis show that the type of dependency is not a significant predictor of depression, nor for three of the four measures of satisfaction. It is, however, a predictor for respondents who reported a great deal of satisfaction with their quality of life. This difference is reflected in the percentage of respondents of VF families reporting a great deal of satisfaction compared with VD, SSD, or IV family respondents.

DISCUSSION AND CONCLUSIONS

Findings from this study show caregivers of children who are technology dependent and receiving home care are predominantly white and middle class. The financial burden and social impact on the family and personal strains vary depending on the type of dependency. Children whose vital functions (VFs) are monitored are the least likely to have developed as other children but are not as much a financial burden and have less social impact and cause less personal strain on the family. Development of children who have specific supportive devices (SSDs) is similar to that of other children. They, too, do not cause financial burden and have less social impact and cause less personal strain on the family. Ventilator-dependent (VD) children and those requiring IV therapy cause financial burden, have a higher social impact, and cause more personal strain on the family than do VF and SSD children.

Depression among caregivers does not vary significantly among the four types of dependencies. Caregivers of IV nutrition or drugs tend to show greater depression than any other group. Depression also seems to be more likely if a child is dependent one or more years.

Satisfaction varies significantly with caregivers. Caregivers who were the least satisfied with care were those with VD children and IV children.

The quality of life for a child who is technology assisted or dependent and their caregivers apparently is affected by persons who work with them in their home. Nurses made up the largest group of professionals who worked with these families. The caregivers expressed that more knowledge was needed about their child's condition and how to care for the child before the child was brought home. There seems to be a need for more definitive discharge planning and teaching of care that family caregivers will be expected to know before the child goes home.

It is likely that more children who are technology dependent will receive care in their home, as it appears that it is more cost-effective. Nurse educators are encouraged to include content in the curriculum that will help future nurses understand how to work with family caregivers in managing children who are technology dependent and cared for at home.

This study is limited in that it could have had more Hispanic caregivers, but a Spanish version of the questionnaire had not been prepared. It is recommended that further studies of children who are technology dependent include a Spanish version so more Hispanic caregivers can participate. The small number of low socioeconomic participants and African American participants suggests that children who are technology dependent in these families may not be cared for in their homes. In future studies about this population of children, every effort should be made to include families that represent the diversity in the population of the country. Follow-up studies on the status of families and these children are encouraged. The implications for longitudinal research on these families and their children who are technology dependent are tremendous. Such studies would add to knowledge about the quality of their lives and their needs.

Follow-up Study

During the year 2000, a follow-up study was conducted of a random sample of the 848 primary care givers of children being cared for in their homes who were technology dependent, and were age 3 months to 19 years when they were interviewed in the early 1990s. A telephone interview using a structured interview guide to determine the status of the children and family was the method used to obtain data. The Internet was used extensively to locate the families as most no longer resided in the homes where they were contacted initially. The findings of the follow-up are described in Chapter 1. Most of the caregivers reviewed children who no longer needed a technology device. Those whose children still needed a device also required professional health care assistance; all of whom except one was a nurse. The children's development academically, behaviorally, and socially compared with children in their own age (the largest number were ranked about average).

REFERENCES

Austin, J. K., & Huberty, T. J. (1989). Revision of the family APGAR for use by 8 year olds. *Family System Medicine, 7*(3), 323–327.

McCubbin, B., & Thompson, N. (Eds.). (1987). *Family assessment inventories for research and practice, family stress coping and health project.* Madison, WI: University of Wisconsin.

McCubbin, H. J., & Patterson, J. M. (1981). *Family stress, resources and coping, Department of Family Social Science.* Minneapolis: University of Minnesota Press.

Office of Technology Assessment. (1987). *Technology dependent children: Home care vs. home care. A technical memorandum.* Washington, DC: Congress of the United States.

Radloff, L. S. (1977). The CES-D Scale: A self-report depression scale for research in the general population. *Applied Psychological Measurement,* (1), 385–401.

Smilkstein, G. (1978). The Family APGAR: A proposal for a family functioning test and its use by physicians. *Journal of Family Practice,* 1231.

Stein, R., & Jessop, D. J. (1984). Does pediatric home care make a difference in children with chronic illness? *Pediatrics, 73,* 545–552.

Stein, R., & Reisman, C. (1982). The development on an impact of family scale: Preliminary findings. *Medical Care, 16,* 465–471.

Part II

Characteristics of Children and Families

Chapter 5

Characteristics of Children

W hat are the characteristics of children who are technology dependent and cared for at home and their families? Most of what
has been published about these children basically reflects that
this population is a special needs group of chronically ill children. Consequently, although such children can be acutely or terminally ill as well,
the information in this chapter will be provided from the perspective of
chronic illness. This, however, does not obviate that much of what is
described may also be applicable to some children who are acutely or
terminally ill.

POPULATION

In 1987, the Office of Technology Assessment (OTA) focused on identifying
children who are technology dependent from the perspective of health
care financing problems. The project was designed to look at existing
evidence on the numbers of technology-dependent children, the relative
cost of home and hospital care, and issues related to how care is financed
(that is how much and exactly what aspects of care are covered by Medicaid
and by insurance) (Office of Technology Assessment, 1987). The child
who is technology dependent was defined by OTA (1987) as one who
needs both a medical device to compensate for the loss of a vital body
function and substantial and ongoing nursing care to avert death or further
disability. The definition was seen as independent of the setting of care or
the particular credentials of the caregiver. As noted in Chapter 1, these
children were classified in four separate population groups and were distinguished from one another by the clinical characteristics unique to the classification.

Many chronically ill children who sometimes require the assistance of
medical devices and frequent nursing care, such as children with hemo-

philia, leukemia and other forms of cancer, diabetes, cystic fibrosis, etc., are likely to increase the overall number of children who are considered technology dependent.

The literature on chronic illness in children is extensive. A brief summary of some of that literature that seems pertinent is provided. Rothenberg and Kaplan (1990) discuss what characterized chronic disease in the 1990s. They note that since 1900 the death rate in the United States had declined by 50% and life expectancy from birth had increased by 27.6 years. Several notions that seem essential to consider in a discussion of health care of children who are chronically ill indicate that we need to recognize that with people living longer, providing needed health care will also occur for a longer period of time for the chronically ill child and his family. The decline in acute, infectious disease and the improvements in treatment have increased the longevity of children with chronic illness (Stein & Jessop, 1984), many of whom are dependent on technology. A partnership between the health care practitioner and the family will be important. Generally, professionals are seen not as individual practitioners but as a part of a system of hospitals, facilities, clinics, schools, and rehabilitation centers. The complexity of the child's condition and the system of services will need to be addressed along with the funding patterns.

Rothenberg and Kaplan (1990) indicate five major program activities that are likely to have a long-term impact on chronic disease. They are screening, community-based programs, preventive medicine, social marketing, and social regulation. While the discussion relative to these activities was given primarily in relationship to conditions associated more with adults, they generally pertain to families and children, particularly those children who are technology dependent and who are cared for by their families at home.

Chronic illness of a child affects the family in varying ways. Information about the effect of chronic illness of a child on families seems to suggest that families that have chronically ill children may experience stress on marital relations, deprivation of leisure time, permanent fatigue, isolation from the community, and financial difficulties (Holoday, 1984; Murphy, 1982). Sabbeth and Leventhal (1984) reviewed 34 studies of marital adjustment on family adjustment to chronic childhood illness. Marital distress was investigated in 83% of the studies. Other areas of marital adjustment, such as communication, decision-making and role flexibility, have received almost no attention.

According to Hobbs, Perrin, and Ireys (1985), much of the research on chronic illness has focused, by necessity, on children seen within only one academic institution. They suggest that interinstitutional studies should be done to allow the pooling of larger numbers of children with given conditions. There is an extensive accumulation of knowledge about children with chronic illness, and the literature on children who are technology dependent is growing. However, many questions remain unanswered. It appears that specialized health care is rarely understood. This may be due in part to a lack of knowledge of the true financial burden imposed by the costs of chronic illness on many families and the primary lack of epidemiological information on the prevalence and the long-term effects and severity of many of those illnesses. This is especially true for those who are technology dependent and cared for in their homes. Hobbs, Perrin, and Ireys (1985) consider cost from the perspectives of identification and evaluation, initial treatment, continuing treatment, special service needs, daily care, and routine costs. Cost is a constant characteristic for almost every parent who has a chronically ill child who is technology dependent. Few data are available to reflect cost specifically on the care of these children. The complexity of the conditions of the children makes it difficult to know and understand the true costs to families.

Technology-dependent children who receive care in the home are viewed as having special needs. These children's special needs may cause undue stress and tax the parents' energy level and ability to handle them if appropriate amounts of support are not provided in a timely manner. In discussing handicapped children whose parents exhaust their energy in caring for them, it has been suggested that such children will not develop to their full potential and may be abused or neglected (Gabarino, 1983; Barth, Blythe, Schinke, & Schilling, 1983). Recognition of respite for parents who have the responsibility for care of technology-dependent children is important.

Vogel and McSkimming (1983) note catheters such as the Hickman are being placed in children for long-term chemotherapy infusions, total parenteral nutrition, blood products, and antibiotics; for obtaining blood samples; and for monitoring central venous pressure. They further note that children with cancer or malabsorption syndromes may have catheters for years. Consequently, the responsibility for catheter care must be transferred to someone in the child's home—usually the parents. They point out the importance of planning and teaching the parents how to care for the catheter.

Kaufman (1985) notes that for ventilator-dependent children, there is a disproportionate emphasis of the home health care plan on medical and advanced technological needs, minimizing the significance of the generic, holistic functions of children and their families. She notes further that three other dimensions are lacking. They are measures to ensure quality of the home care plan, systematic documentation to monitor the ongoing process toward outcome achievement, and information about who will be involved in facilitating achievement outcomes.

Kaufman and Hardy-Ribakow (1987) describe home care as a model of a comprehensive approach for technology-assisted children. More information is needed in the literature related to assessment of developmental and educational needs of these children. Their psychological needs have not been described well, nor has the effect of their illness on other family members been well documented. Reports of community efforts to provide for these children are limited, making program planning difficulty. Although a multidisciplinary approach is important to address the needs of children requiring complex, highly technical care, the role of nursing is critical because much of the care of these children involves nursing. Johnson (1987), in discussing the long-term effects of high technology on the child and family, presents both positives and negatives. She notes that these possible effects may be categorized as physical, psychoemotional, and psychosocial. The child's need for medical technology is an indicator of some loss of physiologic function. The loss may be perceived as a negative. Mobility is important. If a child is not able to move about as is expected in normal development, that child is not likely to perceive the world the same way as one who is mobile. The child sees himself or herself differently and perceives space differently.

From a psychoemotional perspective, Johnson notes that feelings of dehumanization and depersonalization may occur as a result of dependence on machines for human functions basic to life. According to Johnson, stress is the major problem, and the burden of care is overwhelming. Other negative effects that children who are technology dependent may experience are feelings of powerlessness, helplessness, body image problems, negative self-concept, lowered self-esteem, depression, and hopelessness. The child may be socially stigmatized because of the condition of disability. Johnson mentions some positive effects. Among them is a chance for life and improved health because of technology, a sense of control and independence when the child is cared for at home, increased appreciation of life or a deeper spiritual life, and increased family cohesiveness. Baumann (1983) and Rose (1984) discuss vulnerability and coping as concerns of children with chronic conditions. Miller (1983) notes that coping is associated with spiritual well-being.

Fleming (1996), in carrying out further analysis of the 1993 report of her study of 848 children, identifies the characteristics of children who are technology dependent since this population of children seems to be getting more attention in terms of their care. (The basic descriptions of the children and their families are shown in Table 5.1.) See Chapter 4 for more details about how these children are categorized in terms of their dependency on technology.

TABLE 5.1   Descriptions of Technology-Dependent Children and Youth from Fleming Study (1996)

Characteristic	N	%
Gender		
Male	485	57.2
Female	363	42.8
Race		
White	658	77.6
Black	85	10.0
Hispanic	38	4.5
Asian	12	1.4
Native American	14	1.7
Other and mixed races	40	4.7
No response	1	0.1
Residence		
Rural	71	8.4
Small town	197	23.2
Suburbs	253	29.9
City	325	38.3
No response	2	0.2
Number of siblings (under 18 years of age):		
None	254	30.0
1	325	38.3
2	179	21.1
3	49	5.8
4	27	3.2
5 or more	12	1.4
No response	2	0.2
Age		
Under 1 year	216	25.0
1 year to 5 years	427	50.0
6 years to 10 years	121	14.0
11 years to 15 years	52	6.2
16 years and older	32	4.8

Note: The mean age was 4.2 years (SD = 4.5 years).

The primary medical diagnoses of the children by type of dependency are listed in Table 5.2. VD children most frequently had a musculoskeletal or respiratory diagnosis; IV-dependent children had more hematopoietic diagnoses, while SSD-dependent children and VF children most frequently had respiratory diagnoses. However, the children with a respiratory diagnosis in the VD group were in greater need of assistance with respiratory functioning than those in the SSD group. About one in five children overall had a diagnosis of "other," which represents a broad array of conditions, some of which were gastrointestinal, genitourinary, or a multiple-cause diagnosis that did not fit well in the categories.

Because the diagnosis seemed important in describing these children, a separate analysis of the primary diagnoses was done for each type of dependency. The 10 different primary diagnosis categories were very unevenly distributed among the dependency types. In the ventilator-dependent group, most of the children had either an additional respiratory problem and/or an additional feeding problem. The IV-dependent group

TABLE 5.2 Type of Dependency by Primary Diagnosis from Fleming Study (1996)

| Primary Diagnosis | Type of Dependency | | | | | | | | | |
| | Ventilator Dependent | | IV Nutrition or Medication Dependent | | Specific Supportive Device Dependent | | Vital Function Monitoring | | Total | |
	n	%	n	%	n	%	n	%	n	%
Neurological	12	13.3	6	5.1	78	18.4	24	11.1	120	14.2
Respiratory	33	36.7	7	6.0	113	26.6	90	41.8	243	128.6
Cardiac	1	1.1	5	4.3	35	8.2	7	3.3	48	5.7
Metabolic	0	0.0	20	17.1	22	5.2	16	7.4	58	6.9
Endocrine	0	0.0	1	0.9	3	0.7	1	0.5	5	0.6
Renal	0	0.0	2	1.7	7	1.6	12	5.6	21	2.5
Musculoskeletal	34	37.8	4	3.4	59	14.0	4	1.9	101	11.9
Hematopoietic	0	0.0	36	30.8	7	1.6	0	0.0	43	5.1
Genetic	3	3.3	4	3.4	31	4.9	1	0.5	29	3.4
Other	7	7.8	32	27.3	80	18.8	60	27.9	179	21.1
Total	90*	100.0	117	100.0	425	100.0	215	100.0	847	100.0

*One ventilator patient had no primary diagnosis.

was further subdivided into those children who had IV only ($n = 58$) and those who had IV plus some other problem ($n = 59$). Eight others had IVs but were not classified in the IV group because of their primary diagnosis. The SSD-dependent group was easiest to categorize. The four main subgroups were respiratory assistance only ($n = 140$), feeding tubes only ($n = 12$), feeding tubes plus respiratory ($n = 159$), and others ($n = 5$). The VF-dependent group was identified as monitoring device only ($n = 172$), ostomies/urinary catheters ($n = 29$), and all others ($n = 14$).

These findings may have important implications for the OTA classification, considering that OTA apparently did not consider that there was no category that allowed for children who could be placed in more than one group. Some children fit in more than one of OTA's classification. A mixed category may be appropriate. The technology-dependent children cared for in their homes and known to private and public agencies were, as noted in Chapter 2, predominantly white, male, and under 5 years of age. An additional analysis of the primary diagnosis using the four types of dependencies revealed that many of the children in the dependency groups had more than one type of health problem. While these may appear to be random facts they may be of value in understanding this group of children. The importance of recognizing that many of these children had more than one health problem affects the overall classification used by the Office of Technology Assistance.

HELPERS

The percentage of caregivers who relied on someone other than themselves and professionals to help care for their child varied significantly among the four types ($\chi^2(3) = 8.50$, $p = .037$). These individuals were identified as relatives, friends, and others (e.g., neighbors, sitters, etc.). Caregivers of ventilation-dependent children relied on outside help less frequently than caregivers of VF-monitored children (16.5% versus 32.1%). Of the 91 ventilator-dependent children, only 41 caregivers reported that they sought and received help from others in the care of their technology-dependent children. Seventy-three of the 117 IV-dependent, 271 of the 425 SSD-dependent, and 162 of the 215 VF-monitoring caregivers indicated they sought and received help from others in the care of their technology-dependent children. These children and their families are to some extent characterized by the resources they use and need.

PROFESSIONAL SERVICES

Fleming (1993) found in analyzing the data from a study on caregivers and technology-dependent children that 514 of the 848 children she studied were visited by a nurse in their home. The nurse visits were weekly or monthly. In the study it was evident that RN, LPN/LVN, and nursing aides were among the nursing personnel who visited. Some were able to clearly identify the type nurse that visited (most of whom were RNs) and others were not. According to the study, 201 of the nurse visitors (38.2%) assessed, 149 (28.3%) provided support, 101 (19.2%) taught, and 362 (68.8%) provided care to the child. In terms of the equipment, 152 (29.7%) assessed it, 278 (54.3%) serviced the equipment, and 82 (16.8%) did nothing to the equipment. In the other category, 248 (54.3%) provided some type of other service to the family, while 133 (33.3%) provided no other service. In terms of the caregivers, 124 (14.6%) of the 848 had respite service, whereas 724 (85.4%) did not, and 46 (5.4%) used a sitter. Special services included home school and hospice; 24 (28%) of the 848 children received regular schooling at home, and 41 (4.8%) were in preschool. None of the children in the study were receiving hospice care at the time of the investigation.

Children who are technology dependent and being cared for at home by their families are likely to encounter a wide variety of professionals. These professionals must be well educated in several areas. They must know basic physiology and treatment; human growth and development; emotional factors in health and illness; the beliefs, values, and traditions of communities; types of resources; and the ways children learn and school functions. Each professional must be technically proficient in the special skills of his or her own discipline and must have an effective means to maintain and upgrade skills (Hobbs, Perrin, & Ireys, 1985).

PHYSICAL

Of the 848 children in the Fleming (1993) study, 626 (73.8%) had medical supplies or medications, and 754 (88.9%) had medical equipment. It is essential that the medications and equipment needed to deliver care are available. Some children receive nutrition and/or their antibiotics intravenously. Children who need oxygen or who are on apnea monitors or ventilators have to be sure they have the supply of oxygen needed and that the oxygen apparatus and monitors are maintained in good working condition. Children who are dependent on medical devices for proper functioning have specific resource needs (Aradine, 1980; Bloomquist & Lewis-Hunstiga, 1978; DeForest, 1984; Foster & Hoskins, 1981; Frates, Splaingard, Smith, & Harrison, 1985; Loftus, 1988; Vogel & McSkimming, 1983).

Hallam, Rudbeck, and Bradley (1996) found that an increased number of babies born with bronchopulmonary dysphasia need long-term oxygen therapy. The move toward early discharge of these infants to their home was seen as cost saving. What is more important is that these infants can be cared for by their parents in their home. Parsons (1984) notes in her manual that many children dependent on an oxygen apparatus could be reunited with their families earlier if services were available to deliver oxygen. The manual includes criteria for discharge. It delineates specifics for the infant, family, home care coordinator, social workers, and oxygen suppliers.

Advances in medication administration have led to an increase in use of home intravenous therapy as a positive alternative to traditional hospitalization. Sheldon and Bender (1994) note that the transition to home health care for these patients provides a variety of benefits. They specify the criteria for the patient to start home infusion therapy. The criteria should include the following: "(1) an appropriate diagnosis and treatment; (2) a medically stable patient—especially important because patient monitoring in the home is less intensive than in an acute care facility; (3) venous accessibility or a reasonable plan for initiation and maintenance; (4) safe and appropriate home environment, including physical layout, cleanliness, viable telephone access, and electricity; (5) a patient and caregiver capable of being taught and willing to perform necessary care; and (6) financial resources, including the evaluation of all sources, both public and private, to determine scope of home care eligibility" (p. 508).

PSYCHO-EMOTIONAL EFFECTS ON THE CHILD

Mental health difficulties in childhood and early adolescence are best conceptualized as emotions or behaviors outside of the normal range for age and sex and are linked either with an impairment of development/ functioning or with the suffering of the child (Sappitt & Vastanis, 2000). Children who are technology dependent and cared for in the home may exhibit mental health difficulties considering that many of them have chronic health conditions. Psychosocial problems in children who have chronic health conditions have been documented (Cadman, Rosenbaum, & Boyle, 1991).

Emotional development of the child is a continuous process. Erickson's stages of development—the infant (birth to 1 year) develops a sense of trust; the toddler (1 to 3 years) develops a sense of autonomy; the preschooler (3 to 6 years) develops a sense of initiative; the school-age child (6 to 12 years) develops a sense of industry; the early adolescent (12 to 15 years) develops a sense of identity; and the late adolescent (16 to 19 years) develops a sense of intimacy—could be used to help conceptualize and determine if the child is emotionally developing appropriately (Erickson, 1963). The Child Behavior Check List (CBCL) may be a useful tool to assess psychiatric symptoms and social competence; if the child is having home schooling, academic performance can be assessed using the parent-rated version and teacher-rated version (Achenback & Edelbrock, 1983).

Johnson (1987) notes that the imposition of high technology for sustaining vital body function necessitates a significant change in the child's body image. Feelings of dehumanization, depersonalization, loss of freedom, powerlessness, isolation, loss of control and/or privacy, guilt, and depression are some of the psycho-emotional effects that children who are technology dependent may experience. If these feelings persist, it is likely they will affect the child's development negatively. Instead of trust, the infant will develop mistrust; the toddler will develop shame and doubt; the preschooler will develop a sense of guilt; the school-age child will develop a sense of inferiority; the early adolescent will develop diffusion; and the late adolescent a sense of isolation.

The National Mental Health Association launched a public understanding of children's mental health disorders. This association facilitates access to mental health care and helps children with mental health disorders to receive adequate mental health treatment (Sweeney & Neff, 2001). This is very positive, as it is important that services that may result in quality care outcomes for children and their families are promoted. The national evaluation of Comprehensive Community Mental Health Services for children and their families should provide valuable information for those working with children and their families (Holden, Friedman, & Santiago, 2001).

SUMMARY

The characteristics of children presented in this chapter provide some information about children and youth who are technology dependent. New technologies have affected nursing and health care delivery dramatically in the last four decades and, based on the various types of progressive research projects that are being implemented, will continue to do so. The quality of the care of these medically fragile children in their homes in the changing health care environment will likely be a focus. Educators, researchers, and health care providers have an opportunity to be a part of advocating for this vulnerable group of children and their families. Further, the home care market for these children is likely to continue to grow for three reasons, according to Maurano (1994). They are

1. an increased survivorship of very low birth weight children as a result of advances in medical technology;
2. greater longevity for children with terminal illness; and
3. greater awareness and detection of chronic health problems by parents, educators, and physicians.

REFERENCES

Achenback, T., & Edelbrock, C. (1983). *Manual for the child behavior check list and revised child profile.* Burlington, VT: Department of Psychiatry, University of Vermont.

Aradine, C. (1980). Home care for young children with long-term tracheotomies. *Maternal Child Nursing, 5,* 121–125.

Barth, R. R., Blythe, B. J., Schinke, S. P., & Schilling, R. R. (1983). Self-control training with maltreating parents. *Child Welfare, 62,* 313–324.

Baumann, R. R. (1983). Coping behavior of children experiencing powerlessness from loss of mobility. In J. F. Miller (Ed.), *Coping with chronic illness: Overcoming powerlessness.* Philadelphia: F. A. Davies.

Bloomquist, L., & Lewis-Hunstiga, M. J. (1978). To care for the child at home: Discharge planning for the child with leukemia. *Cancer Nursing,* 303–308.

Butler, P., Englebrecht, R. E., Tait, J. H., Stallard, J., & Patrick, J. H. (1985). Physiological cost index of walking for normal children and its use as an indicator of physical handicap. *Developmental Medicine Child Neurology, 26*(5), 607–612.

Cadman, D., Rosenbaum, P., & Boyle, M. (1991). Children with chronic illness: Family and parent demographic characteristics and psychosocial adjustment. *Pediatrics, 87,* 884–889.

DeForest, J. (1984). Home apnea monitoring in infancy. *Canadian Nurse, 80*(5), 37–41.

Erickson, E. H. (1963). *Childhood and society.* New York: W. W. Norton.

Fleming, J. (1996). Characteristics of high-tech home care of technology dependent children. Unpublished report, College of Nursing, University of Kentucky, Lexington.

Fleming, J. (1993). *Home care of technology dependent children resources.* Unpublished report, College of Nursing, University of Kentucky, Lexington.

Foster, S., & Hoskins, D. Home care of child with a tracheotomy tube. *Pediatric Clinics of North America*, 28(4), 855–857.

Frates, R. C., Splaingard, M. I., Smith, E. O., & Harrison, G. M. (1985). Outcome of home mechanical ventilation in children. *Journal of Pediatrics*, 106, 850–856.

Gabarino, J. (1983). What do we know about child maltreatment? *Children and Youth Services Review*, 5, 3–6.

Hallam, L., Rudbeck, B., & Bradley, M. (1996). Resource use and costs of caring for oxygen dependent children: A comparison of hospital home based care. *Journal of Neonatal Nursing*, 2(2), 25–30.

Hobbs, J., Perrin, J. M., & Ireys, H. T. (1985). *Chronically ill children and their families.* San Francisco: Jossey-Bass.

Holden, E. W., Friedman, R. M., & Santiago, R. L. (2001). Overview of the National Evaluation of the Comprehensive Mental Health Services for Children and Their Families Program. *Journal of Emotional and Behavioral Disorders*, 9(1), 4.

Holoday, B. (1984). Challenges of rearing a chronically ill child. *Nursing Clinics of North America*, 19, 361–368.

Johnson, D. L. (1987). Possible long-term effects of high technology on the child and family. *Focus on Critical Care*, 14(4), 43–50.

Kaufman, (1985). Private communication.

Kaufman, J., & Hardy-Ribakow, D. (1987). Home care: A model of a comprehensive approach for technology assisted chronically ill children. *Journal of Pediatric Nursing*, 2, 244–249.

Loftus, T. (1988). Helping cystic fibrosis patients with high-tech home care. *Caring*, 7, 22–27.

Maurano, L. W. (1994). Community and home care. In C. L. Betz, M. Hunsberger, & S. Wright (Eds.), *Family-centered nursing care of children* (2nd ed.). Philadelphia: W. B. Saunders.

Miller, J. F. (1983). *Coping with chronic illness: Overcoming powerlessness.* Philadelphia: F. A. Davis.

Murphy, M. A. (1982). The family with a handicapped child: A review of literature. *Journal of Developmental Behavioral Pediatrics*, 5(2), 73–82.

Office of Technology Assessment. (1987). *Technology dependent children: Hospital vs. home care—a technical memorandum* (OTA-TM-H-38). Washington, DC: U.S. Government Printing Office.

Parsons, C. (1984). Manual on home oxygen for infants: A discharge planning guide. *Critical Care Nurse*, 84–85.

Pless, I. B. (1974). Theoretical and practical consideration in the measurement of outcomes. In D. G. Gilman & I. B. Pless (Eds.), *Chronic Childhood Illness: Assessment of Outcome. A Conference sponsored by the John E. Forgarty International Center for Advanced Study in the Health Sciences and the National Institutes of Health.* Bethesda, MD: U.S. Department of Health, Education and Welfare.

Rose, M. H. (1984). The concepts of coping and vulnerability as applied to children with chronic conditions. *Issues Comprehensive Pediatric Nursing*, 7, 177–186.

Rothenberg, R. B., & Kaplan, J. P. (1990). Chronic disease in the 1990's. *Annual Review of Public Health*, 11, 267–296.

Sabbeth, B., & Leventhal, J. (1984). Marital adjustment to chronic childhood illness: A critique of literature. *Pediatrics, 73,* 762–768.

Sappitt, R., & Vastanis, R. (2000). Children and adolescents' difficulties. In Newell & Gowmay (Eds.), *Mental health nursing* (pp. 313–330). New York: Churchill Livingstone.

Sheldon, P., & Bender, M. (1994). High Tech Home Care: An Overview of Intravenous Therapy. *Nursing Clinics of North America, 29*(3), 507–519.

Sheldon, P., & Bender, M. (1994). High technology in home care: An overview of intravenous therapy. *Nursing Clinics of North America, 29*(8), 507–579.

Stein, R., & Jessop, D. J. (1984). Does pediatric home care make a difference for children with chronic illness? Findings from Pediatric Ambulatory Care Treatment Study. *Pediatrics, 73,* 845–853.

Sweeney, R., & Neff, M. (2001). NMHA launches a campaign for children's mental health. *American Family Physician, 63*(12), 2319.

Vogel, T. C., & McSkimming, S. A. (1983). Teaching parents to give indwelling c.v. catheter care. *Nursing, 83,* 55–56.

Chapter 6

Characteristics of Families

Families are the nurturing centers of human development and the primary agents in health. Further, the family can be the best bulwark for good mental health in that ties of affection and intimacy can be established. It can provide individual members with personal security and acceptance; satisfaction and a sense of purpose; companionship; and limit setting. Finally, the family promotes the culture as it begins the acculturation process that, as the child grows and develops, is promoted by other agencies in the society.

The contemporary nurse who provides care to technology-dependent children cannot overlook the importance of the family as a vital resource. It facilitates viewing the family from a holistic perspective and enables one to form a partnership with the family and to respect the unique characteristics that the family as a group presents, as well as individual members of the group, and their effect on the child.

Research into family environment and development is important in determining characteristics. A few select references, which seem to be pertinent to this matter, are highlighted. Bronfenbrenner (1977) considered development from an ecological perspective with specific reference to the social and cultural context in which it occurs. The child and the family's ecological and cultural world (ecocultural) are defined by the immediate setting—the home and the major institutions or agencies as they directly or indirectly affect them.

Nursing practice is dependent on (1) having some conceptualization of the characteristics of the children who are technology dependent and their families; (2) enhancement of knowledge and relevant nursing skills in the effective and appropriate use of the technologies; and (3) recognition that many parents prefer home care to a hospital stay for their children who are technology dependent. In order to provide effective home care of high quality, the family will need

- adequate training and preparation
- appropriate and well-maintained equipment

- adequate social and psychological support services
- proper transportation
- availability in the community of emergency facilities
- competent case management service
- high-quality respite care service

RESOURCES

Family, financial, community, professional, and physical resources are essential for children who are technology dependent and cared for at home and their families. Home care that combines the latest in medical technology with traditional comfort and security requires services and products in the home limited only by the imagination of medical equipment, research, and design experts and the willingness of home care personnel to provide the services (Haddad, 1996). Limits do exist, such as the availability of reimbursement for services and products, the capabilities of patients and families, and the very real problem of providing care in an environment that was not originally designed for this purpose. Resources in the form of services such as those available in the community and from professionals, and products in the form of medicine and equipment are vital in providing quality health care to children who are technology dependent and receiving care in their home. The outcome of care is dependent on having finances that make it possible to have these resources available.

Information provided in this section may help professionals to create projects in their communities and/or to stimulate ideas for research studies or innovative means to assist families with resources in their practice.

Family-centered care in pediatric nursing is essential, as it acknowledges the fact that most children live in families and that the family is critical in molding their lives. As the trends in health care in society change and the populations that are cared for by health professionals become more diverse in terms of their race and ethnicity, the more vital the family and family environment becomes. This is particularly true for caregiving families who provide complex health care in their homes.

Research on the effects of the family environment on the development of children is extensive. Feetham (1984) has delineated concepts about families that are progressive and timely. The concepts were characteristics of the family such as role, structure, communication patterns, coping, and internal and external functioning of the family. Although most researchers agree that family environment has incredible power to facilitate development, there is no consensus as to what the variables are (Zajonc, 1976). The family as a system is seen as organizationally complex—that is, a collection of entities interconnected by a complex network of relationships (Kantor & Lehr, 1975). The family network from a systems perspective is open, adaptive, and information processing. Open means that there are both internal and external interchanges that can be redefined, depending on what the focus is in the system at any one time. Strategies that the family uses are rational and purposeful.

The contention of the author is that if nurses wish to improve care to children, a greater awareness of sociocultural factors of family dynamics and the contemporary aspects of family life is necessary. Accurate assessments of the family are essential in planning, implementing, and delivering care. Understanding the strengths and weaknesses of the family, interpersonal relationships, roles, the developmental level of the family, and the competency of the family provide baseline information as well as present a definitive picture of the family with whom the nurse was working.

WHAT IS A FAMILY?

A broad definition of family is a group of two or more persons joined by ties of marriage, blood, or adoption, who constitute a single household, who interact with each other in their respective familial roles, and who create and maintain a common culture (Winch, 1952). Consequently, a child may be a member of

- a single-parent family (mother or father and children). This type of family seems on the increase;
- a nuclear family (mother, father, and children). This type of family seems to be decreasing;
- an extended family (mother, father, children, and other relatives, such as grandparents);
- an expanded family that may be a combination of kinship arrangements (mother, aunt, and children; father, cousins, and children; grandparents, mother, and children, etc.)
- an aggregate family or blended family (divorced people who marry and each bring children to the new marriage).

The family unit with children may be composed of divorced parents, widowed parents, unmarried parents, adoptive parents, foster-home parents, institutional surrogate parents, or stepparents. Contemporary families are indeed diverse and varied.

The various combinations of relationships in families with children are numerous. The one basic factor, however, when children are involved is that someone in the family assumes the parenting role. The role of being a parent in the modern-day world is not easy. The assumption of the parenting role might well be described as a situational crisis. Only in recent years has the subject of parenthood been regarded as one worthy of careful study and preparation. Somerville (1972) states, "Despite the importance attached to parenthood in the society, there is little serious effort to prepare young people for the responsibility. Many young parents are ill-prepared for the physical and psychological inroads on time, energy, finances, and relationships which the coming of children brings" (pp. 121–122). The issues of parenting, according to Chinn (1974), range in kind and complexity from the initial stages of parenthood immediately postpartum to ongoing processes such as teaching and assisting parents to provide adequate nutrition for a growing family, or helping a family achieve effective discipline and emotional security.

CONCEPTUAL FRAMEWORKS FOR ASSESSING FAMILIES

Families, like individuals, need to be assessed. They are not what they may appear to be on first impression. In assessing families to plan nursing care to children, some frameworks for viewing the family, which will enhance nurses' understanding of sociocultural factors in the family, may be used, as described below.

Family Strengths and Weaknesses

"Strengths are defined as those factors which contribute to family unity and solidarity and that foster the development of the potentials inherent within the family" (Otto, 1963, p. 88). Weaknesses, of course, would be those factors that mitigate against unity and solidarity and that do not foster development. The strands of a framework that consider strengths and weaknesses of the family are

- physical, emotion, and spiritual needs of the family
- child rearing practices and discipline

- communication
- support, security, and encouragement
- growth producing relationships and experience within and outside the family
- community relationships
- growth of parents with children
- self-help and accepting help
- flexibility of family functions and roles
- mutual respect for individuality
- family unit, loyalty, and intrafamily cooperation
- flexibility of family strengths

Planning and implementing care for a child in a family using a strength-and-weakness framework is likely to force the nurse to view the family and the child realistically. If objective appraisal is done, the nurse sees not only problems and negative features of the family but also assets and positive features.

Role Theory

A "role" is the part played by the individual in the family. Roles may be seen as primary mechanisms serving essential functioning prerequisites in governing human behavior. Interactionists see role as focusing on behavior, in which the acts and symbols of the individuals who are interacting have for each other.

Every individual in the family occupies a role. Each individual functions in or occupies several roles. The child, for example, may be a male, a son, a brother, a student, and so on. The underlying concept in role theory is that of complementarity of roles. Roles do not exist in isolation but are situated to relate to that of a role partner. In considering role difficulties, Rapport and Rosow (1966) note three factors that must be considered: the position in which the failure occurs, the social norm or behavior expected, and the personality of the individual.

Recognition of role in the interactive process by nurses who provide care is essential. Role choice of mothers and fathers in our changing society should be accepted by health care professionals as rights of the individual. Interest in parent-child relationships may be on the increase, rather than only mother-child relationships. Research studies in the past few decades of the father-infant attachment and relationships seems to suggest that the traditional roles assumed by mother and father may be changing. The change reflects a greater valuing of the father's role in the child's early development. Lynn (1974) identifies factors that have contributed to the "undermining" of the father's role. Some of these are (1) the father's absence and detachment because of work demands; (2) knowledge explosion and rapidity of change, making it hard for fathers to keep up with their children's knowledge level; (3) divorce; and (4) the changing nature of sex roles. Concern with the consistency of roles among family members and norms in actual role performance, the compatibility of the roles and norms within the community norms, and the ability of the family to meet the psychological needs of the members of the family group as well as its ability to respond to change will aid in making assessments of the adequacy of family functioning. Nurses using a framework that considers role would likely be inclined to support the father's role in parenting as well as the mother's.

Interactional Theory

A third framework of family, which might be useful to nurses providing care to technology-dependent children, is interactional theory. This framework is a system designed to view the personal relationships between husband and wife and parents and children as interacting personalities. The relationships between mates and between children and parents are viewed as dynamic. In this context, interaction means that the behavior of one individual is the cause and effect of the behavior of others. The nurse who uses this framework will likely be able to focus on how members of the family are influenced and how decisions are made. The dynamics that enter into interactions might also be determined.

Developmental Approaches

A fourth framework is the family development approach, in which there are orderly sequential changes to be expected in growth, development, and dissolution within families throughout the entire family cycle. Strands of this framework consider

1. Social time: The life cycle of the nuclear family, beginning with expanding families, child-rearing families, preschool, teenage, contracting families, and families launching young adults. Middle-age parents also are considered.

2. Structure: The family group of interacting individuals, and its development over time.
3. Configuration: Life cycle, stages, and family tempo.
4. Cohesion: Developmental tasks of family members.
5. Conditions: Teachable movements and psychological elements, such as perception, identity formation, and motivation.
6. Overt behaviors: Are both transactional and interactional for the adult parent and the child. Each responds based on the overt behaviors they encounter. All of these strands play a role in not only the child's development but the adults and the family's development.

A related conceptual framework is the family life cycle, a framework that looks at the family as it develops in stages over a period of time. Duvall (1971) describes eight stages of the family life cycle: early marriage and expectant family, childbearing family (birth to 30 months), preschool family ($2^{1}/_{2}$ to 5 years), school-age family (5 to 12 years), family with teenagers (13 to 19 years), family as launching center (early 20s), the aging family, and families in crisis. The family life cycle, as described by Duvall, has two states—the expanding family stage, which takes the family from its inception to the time the children are grown, and the contracting family stage, where the children are being launched by the family to live their lives. In stages two through five, children are included as members of the family. Their ages are key to determining the state of the family.

Duvall (1977) identifies family development tasks as

1. providing shelter, food, clothing, health care, etc. for family members;
2. meeting family costs and allocating such resources as time, space, facilities, etc., according to each member's need;
3. determining who does what in the support, management, and care of the home and its members;
4. ensuring each member's socialization through the internalization of increasingly mature roles in the family and beyond;
5. establishing ways of interacting, communicating, expressing affection, aggression, sexuality, etc. within limits acceptable to society; and
6. bearing (or adopting) and rearing children, and incorporating and releasing family members.

Duvall indicates that all families have these basic tasks as long as they exist. They perform the tasks in their own ways. Families in various ethnic, racial, and social class groupings operate within the freedoms and constraints of their subcultures as well as those of the larger society. The nurse could easily use Duvall's framework and development tasks in assessing the family regardless of sociocultural background, as they clearly delineate the stages and tasks of the family.

ASSESSING FAMILY FUNCTIONING

The frameworks above are rather basic ways the nurse can view families from a sociocultural perspective. Other means for conceptualizing the family, which may enhance a perspective of sociocultural dimensions, follow. Basically, each describes families in different states of crises or malfunctions, as well as a families that are adequately adjusted or adapted.

A final framework considers the family's ability to cope. Hill and Hansen (1960, 1964) identified four interrelated but conceptually distinct factors that influence the family's ability to cope with the illness experience. they are characteristics of the event; perceived threat to family relationships, status, and goals; resources available to the family; and past experience with the same or similar situations.

Lewis (1980), in describing typical families, reflects the quality of family life at different points on what is called a continuum of family competence.

1. Optimal families are viewed basically as families with high levels of psychological maturity. These families negotiate in solving problems. Their communications are clear, and members of the family assume responsibility for their thoughts and actions. Children are accomplishing age-appropriate developmental tasks.
2. Competent but pained families are viewed as less well adapted as optimal families. The wife in these families seems angry and unhappy. She feels deprived of her husband's affection and often forms coalitions with an individual who appears to function as an ally. Sometimes this alliance is with a child. The husband recognizes the wife's unhappiness but is generally not empathetic.
3. Dysfunctional families are viewed as basically two types: the dominant-submissive family and the chronically conflicted one. In the dominant-submissive family, either the wife or the husband is dominant and the other submissive. In the chronically conflicted family, each parent tries to dominate the other. They do not share power. These families do not negotiate in solving problems; they deny

problems. Severely dysfunctional families are the least competent and do not support maturation and growth for the parents or the children.

ECONOMIC CONSIDERATIONS

When assessing, planning, and implementing care to children in the family, nurses need to ensure that they get information that will provide an index of economic status—information regarding social and environmental deprivation. Knowledge of the composition of the family, mean occupancy per room, water supply, sanitation facilities, and adequacy of the kitchen should be determined if continuity of care in the home is expected. Information relating to the child's past medical history and current state of health is important. Development of the child also is essential. Information regarding nutritional status of the child and his/her family is important in preventing, screening, and following up potential problems.

In making the assessment, it would be desirable for nurses to consider the concept of anticipatory guidance as very important when planning with families. Iorio (1968) noted that anticipatory guidance provides parents with much of what to expect and what to do about it, which ultimately strengthens the parenthood role. The assessment will aid the nurse in obtaining objective data not only on parental interactions but also on siblings and other members of the family.

The above frameworks or modification of them may be useful in assessing families. Since the family is an important resource in managing care for children who are technology dependent, having a base or structure on which to make observations is likely to enhance the nurse's objectivity in approach and in developing strategies of care regardless of the sociocultural background of the family with whom the nurse works. Once the plans for care are made, they can be continually checked.

Family-oriented, community-based care of children who are technology dependent needs resources to provide competent care to the children. Knoll (1992) captures the dilemma in which families find themselves. He notes that the official rhetoric affirms the primacy of the family, but the experience of families is otherwise.

There is evidence to suggest that the present budgeting system has profound implications for the number and quality of nurses working in home care. Many successful nurses are becoming entrepreneurs or leaving nursing and are no longer available for service in public agencies. Consequently, many of those left to serve the public agencies do not have adequate public health nursing background or adequate technical skills needed to provide "high tech" care. Further, they may need a more adequate support system to reinforce their commitment to the delivery of high-quality care and case management.

THE IMPACT OF A TECHNOLOGY-DEPENDENT CHILD ON THE FAMILY

A few brief reports of studies that consider some specific characteristics of families with children who are technology dependent are presented. A descriptive study of the characteristics and the coping patterns of families with infants on home apnea monitoring revealed significant correlations among family functioning scores and coping patterns subscale scores. McCaleb and Luther (1996) conducted this study to describe the characteristics of families with children who required apnea monitors in the home setting. The families of 22 children ranging in age from 8 to 64 months were studied. Findings indicate that the families were high in adaptability and average in cohesion. Findings support the importance of understanding the role of family functioning and coping patterns of families with children on home apnea monitoring.

S. B. Reed (1991), in addressing the consequences that cystic fibrosis has on a family unit, notes that it is vital that nurses are able to differentiate between a family having difficulty coping with a child with cystic fibrosis in the home and one that is coping well on its own. The children of families that are not coping well tend to be hospitalized more than those of families coping well. This characteristic is reflected in the family's use of the hospital. They tend to use the hospitalizations as rest periods for themselves. By recognizing the clues of a family having problems, early intervention can and should be initiated before the family is in crisis.

Noncompliance with Medical Regimen

Tebbi (1993) reports finding a significant noncompliance with self-administered medication, especially in chronic conditions such as cancer. The characteristic of noncompliance transcends the boundary of disease categories and age groups. Noncompliance, however, is most prevalent during adolescent years, when the process of transition from parental dependency to autonomy produces confusion as to who is responsible for administration of medication. Administration of parenteral medications in the home is possible with the availability of venous access ports and easy to operate pumps. This adds another dimension to the self-administration of medication that previously concerned mainly oral therapy. Various factors including treatment characteristics determine how well a given regimen is adhered to. Because of the number of determinants (e.g., the patient, disease, health care providers, and, as noted above, treatment characteristics), it is not always possible to identify noncompliers or to predict the level of patient adherence to treatment with any degree of certainty. Compliance is a complex issue. Family and social support, individualized programs, reminders to reduce forgetfulness, personalized needs assessment, and education are identified by Tebbi as some approaches that can reduce noncompliance.

IMPACT OF CAREGIVING

How parents and siblings cope is important. Most families need help with providing care in the home to a child who has used a medical device and/ or nursing care to perform physiological body functions. Some specific information as to the impact on helping the family adapt and cope is highlighted in the portion of the chapter.

A description of the primary caregivers of the 848 children reported by Fleming (1996) are in Table 6.1. Fleming et al. (1994) compared the impact on the family of the four categories of children who are technology dependent using the Impact on Family Scale (Stein & Reissman, 1980) and the Center for Epidemiological Studies Depression Scale (CES-D). They found a significant difference among the four types of technology dependency for impact on the family. They found that socioeconomic status had a significant effect on depressive symptoms of families with a child dependent on a medical device and cared for in the home. They also found that children whose vital functions were monitored were the least likely to have developed as other children but were not as much a financial burden nor did they socially affect or cause personal strains on the family. Other findings of impact on the 848 caregivers studied by Fleming et al. are indicated in Tables 6.2–6.12.

FAMILY COPING

The impact of home care on specific conditions and uses of technology are noted here to provide perspective on what families experience with

TABLE 6.1   Description of the Primary Caregiver

Characteristic	N	%
Relationship to child		
Mother	745	87.9
Father	37	4.4
Adoptive parent	29	3.4
Foster parent	18	2.1
Other	19	2.2
Age of caregiver		
17 to 24	83	9.8
25 to 34	418	49.3
35 to 44	287	33.8
45 to 54	50	5.9
55 to 65	10	1.2
Marital status		
Married	650	76.7
Divorced	52	6.1
Separated	40	4.7
Never married	57	6.7
Remarried	14	1.7
Widowed	12	1.4
Did not respond	23	2.7
Educational level		
Last grade completed		
Less than 12th	88	10.4
12th grade	271	32.1
1 year of college	78	9.2
2 years of college	131	15.4
3 years of college	50	5.9
4 years of college	130	15.3
Greater than 4 years of college	100	11.7
Religious preference		
Protestant	393	46.3
Catholic	283	33.4
Jewish	24	2.8
None	67	8.0
Other	81	9.5
Work status		
Working outside the home	353	41.6
Not working outside the home	495	58.4
Annual family income		
Under $25,000	284	33.5
$25,000 to $50,000	333	39.3
Over $50,000	207	24.4
No response	24	2.8

Responses given by caregivers on the impact that caring for a child who is technology dependent has on the family are indicated in Tables 6.1 to 6.12. Source: Fleming's study of 848 technology-dependent children.

TABLE 6.2   Response to Statement, "Nobody Understands the Burden I Carry"

Response	N	%
Strongly agree	106	12.5
Agree	264	31.1
Disagree	395	46.6
Strongly disagree	43	5.1
Not sure	39	4.6
Do not know	1	0.1

TABLE 6.3   Response to Statement, "Traveling to the Hospital Is a Strain on Me"

Response	N	%
Strongly agree	148	17.5
Agree	380	44.8
Disagree	288	34.0
Strongly disagree	16	1.9
Not applicable	13	1.5
Not sure	2	0.2
Do not know	1	0.1

TABLE 6.4   Response to Statement, "Sometimes I Feel Like We Live on a Roller-Coaster in Crisis When My Child Is Ill, Okay When Things Are Stable"

Response	N	%
Strongly agree	354	41.7
Agree	350	41.3
Disagree	121	14.3
Strongly disagree	6	0.7
Not sure	16	1.9
Do not know	1	0.1

TABLE 6.5   Response to Statement, "It Is Hard to Find a Reliable Person to Take Care of the Child When You Need Help"

Response	N	%
Strongly agree	268	31.6
Agree	316	37.3
Disagree	222	26.2
Strongly disagree	22	2.6
Not applicable	15	1.8
Not sure	1	0.1
Do not know	4	0.5

TABLE 6.6   Response to Statement, "I Live from Day to Day and Do Not Plan for the Future"

Response	N	%
Strongly agree	124	14.6
Agree	303	35.7
Disagree	353	41.6
Strongly disagree	46	5.4
Not sure	20	2.4
Do not know	2	0.2

TABLE 6.7   Response to Statement, "Fatigue Is a Problem for Me Because of Child's Illness"

Response	N	%
Strongly agree	173	20.4
Agree	381	44.9
Disagree	263	31.0
Strongly disagree	13	1.5
Not sure	18	2.1

TABLE 6.8   Response to Statement, "Learning to Manage My Child's Illness Has Made Me Feel Better"

Response	N	%
Strongly agree	165	19.5
Agree	558	65.8
Disagree	74	8.7
Strongly disagree	5	0.6
Not sure	41	4.8
Do not know	5	0.6

TABLE 6.9   Response to Statement, "Because of What We Have Shared, We Are a Better Family"

Response	N	%
Strongly agree	203	23.9
Agree	408	56.6
Disagree	79	9.3
Strongly disagree	13	1.5
Not applicable	59	7.0
Not sure	6	0.7
Do not know	8	0.9

TABLE 6.10   Response to Statement, "My Partner and I Discuss My Child's Problems Together"

Response	N	%
Strongly agree	197	23.3
Agree	501	59.2
Disagree	65	7.7
Strongly disagree	16	1.9
Not sure	11	1.3
Not applicable	55	6.5
Do not know	2	0.1

TABLE 6.11   Response to Statement, "I Try to Treat My Child as if He/ She Were a Normal Child"

Response	N	%
Strongly agree	215	25.4
Agree	560	66.0
Disagree	48	5.7
Strongly disagree	5	0.6
Not applicable	15	1.8
Not sure	2	0.2
Do not know	3	0.4

TABLE 6.12   Response to Statement, "My Relatives Have Been Understanding and Helpful with My Child"

Response	N	%
Strongly agree	200	23.6
Agree	468	55.2
Disagree	109	12.9
Strongly disagree	35	4.1
Not applicable	22	2.6
Not sure	10	1.2
Do not know	4	0.5

children who are technology dependent (Thorne, Radford, & Armstrong, 1977). Findings from a longitudinal study of families caring for a child with a gastronomy revealed a complex set of coping strategies that were effective. A national survey in Sweden of children receiving home parenteral nutrition revealed that families appeared to have adapted well, that linear growth was normal for the children, and that the school-age child attended age-relevant level classes (Carlsson, Hakansson, Rubensson, & Finkel, 1997). Vandvik and Eckblad (1991) report that of 84 mothers interviewed as a part of a longitudinal project of mothers of children with a recent onset of rheumatic disease, 50% reported psychiatric distress. Associations were made with maternal distress, psychosocial variables, and the disease of the child. Trait anxiety was unrelated to disease variables but was associated with psychosocial background variables.

Quint, Chesterman, Crain, Winkleby, and Boyce (1990) studied the impact of providing home care for ventilator-dependent children in a cross-sectional survey of 18 Northern California families. They used the Impact on Family Scale and found no differences in the perceived family impact between primary caretakers and their spouses. Primary caretakers in the sample, however, showed significantly reduced coping subscale scores with a longer duration of home ventilatory care.

A 7-year demonstration pilot project of adult and pediatric long-term ventilator-dependent children conducted by Kaiser Permanente from 1985 to 1992 was designed to investigate if home care was a realistic alternative to continued hospital care (Baldwin-Meyers & Oppenheimer, 1996). It is interesting to note that the perceptions of patients and others providing direct care in regard to health status, life satisfaction, emotional well-being, caregiver ability, and professional care and services found the quality of care at home was similar to hospital care. Quality of life was judged to be better at home.

After describing factors predicting maternal adjustments in mothers caring for medical fragile infants, Miles, Holditch-Davis, Burchinal, and Nelson (1999) conclude that nurses should consider personal characteristics and level of parental role attainment. They also conclude that the characteristics of the child and illness-related distress in their approaches to intervention with the mothers of these infants should be considered. These investigators collected data for their longitudinal study at hospital discharge and at 6, 12, and 16 months after the child's birth.

"Living in a house of cards" was a phenomenon described by O'Brien (2001) in addressing families' experiences who are providing long-term home care for children who are technology dependent. Families cited frequent change, uncertainty, and unpredictability in their lives. To increase stability, the use of vigilance, advocacy, and reframing were used. The main problems with pediatric home ventilation in Switzerland, according to Hammer (2000), are its negative psychosocial impact on family life, limited home care resources, financial burden, differences in ethical perception by the local community, and the fact that the equipment is usually designed for adults. Beresford (1982) found that parents had a wide range of coping strategies that they employed with enormous creativity to deal with the problems they faced in caring for a severely disabled child. Siegel, Raveis, Houts, and Mor (1991) studied caregiver burden. Four hundred eighty-three patients with cancer and their informal caregivers were studied. In general, the unmet needs of the caregiver decreases as the domains of assistance provided by the caregiver increases.

Dimagio and Sheetz (1983) found that the stressors associated with a child's illness that result in family disruption depend on the nature, severity, length, and prognosis of the illness and on the parents' coping ability. Specifically, they depend on the family's support systems, financial resources, educational background, previous experience with illness, and a variety of individual differences. It's perhaps trite to state that the impact on the family is likely to be different for each family. The general statement that can be made is that anxiety is a normal reaction of a family to illness and should be expected.

Kiernan (1995) substantiates the position of the investigators above in her study of families of chronically ill children dependent upon home IV therapy. She found that the burden imposed with the use of IV technology added to the stress of chronic health problems. She also found stress related to the imposition of health care providers in the home. It is interesting, however, to note that despite added stress, respondents in her study were more satisfied with family life and had more well-being than the normative sample. She also reports higher family cohesion scores than in a normative sample.

Campbell (1998) uses a case study to describe the special needs of a technology-dependent child and the impact of chronic illness on both child and family. According to Campbell, children who are technology dependent and cared for at home present unique challenges for families and health professionals. The financial, social, and emotional capacities of parents are stretched because of the medical and nursing needs of these children.

Family social status can account for significant variation both before and after the discharge of children who are technology dependent to the home and to community-based care, according to the findings of Cohen (1999), who studied the transition of these children from discharge planning to 1 year following discharge. Theoretical relationships between family social status and the concepts of moral distress and social trajectory were found.

The stresses experienced by families caring for children who are technology dependent have been documented well. The resilience of many families who care for these children is remarkable. It is remarkable how well many families have been able to cope with the situations in which they find themselves. Caring for a child who is technology dependent at home can affect the family negatively and positively. Fleming et al. (1994) report that the high depression group in their study had greater intrafamily strains and marital strains. Families gave up things because of the ill child. In spite of factors such as fatigue and an inability to leave the home because a reliable person to care for the child could not be found, 90% of the families reported that learning to manage their child's illness made them feel better about themselves. They also reported overwhelmingly that because of what the family shared, they were a better family.

Following are some intervention strategies that need to be addressed to help minimize negative impact of stressors on the family:

1. Assuring effective discharge planning (Cohen, 1999).
2. Recognizing the uniqueness of each child who is technology dependent and his/her family.
3. Determining with families their priorities (Feinberg, 1999).
4. Educating families as to how to deliver care (Feinberg, 1999).
5. Engaging in activities that increase the stability of family (O'Brien, 2001).
6. Recognizing areas of change (O'Brien, 2001).
7. Supporting families based on the needs indicated.
8. Identifying community services available to assist and support families and preparing for respite care as need indicates.
9. Recognizing the importance of coordination of care and facilitating coordination of care.

CAREGIVERS IN THE FLEMING STUDY

Fleming (1996), in a report on the 848 primary caregivers of children who were technology dependent studied, identifies the characteristics of families of home-based children who are technology dependent. As noted in Chapter 4, a geographic sample was obtained from 13 cities which served as the data collection areas. Criteria for sample selection of the caregivers were that: (1) they were receiving care from a public or private agency; (2) the children for whom they cared must have received care at least 1 month in the home; and (3) the children were between the ages of 3 months and 19 years. This age group was selected because it covers infants through the adolescent years. To avoid bias and logistical problems, a three-stage sampling procedure was used to select the participants for the study. Descriptions of the conceptual model, the sampling technique, instrument, the procedure for the study, and data analysis are provided in Chapter 4.

The basic description of the characteristics of caregivers of children is shown in Table 6.1. Most families of the children in this study owned a vehicle (86.0%, *n* = 729). A few (7.3%, *n* = 62) relied on some form of public transportation, friends/relatives (3.4%, *n* = 29), or other means to transport the children to medical care providers.

Financing Care

Caregivers were asked to identify from a list of payment choices how medical bills were paid. Private health insurance was the response of 524 (61.8%), Medicaid for 331 (39.0%), HMO/PPO for 88 (10.4%) and family donations for 53 (6.3%) of the responders. Several of the respondents listed more than one source.

In response to a statement that the illness caused financial problems for the family, 172 (20.3%) strongly agreed, 306 (36.1%) agreed, 323 (38.1%) disagreed, 33 (3.9%) strongly disagreed, and 15 (1.8%) were not sure. Over 60% of the caregivers indicated they lost time from work because of hospital or clinic appointments for the children.

Caregiver Perception

Professionals who worked with families in the home were mostly public health nurses. Four hundred fifty-seven children (53.9%) were visited by RNs, and 185 (21.8%) were visited by LPNs/LVNs. Of those who had nursing visits, 470 (55.4%) caregivers indicated that they were pleased with the way the nurse cared for their child. Seventy-five (8.8%) indicated the visiting nurse was a case manager for the child's care while 389 (45.8%) indicated they had a nursing manager. Caregivers were satisfied with their own care of the child and seemed to use nurses primarily for information and demonstration of care. More than 80% of the caregivers indicated a need for information about how to care for their technology-dependent children when asked what they felt caregivers needed most.

When caregivers were asked what was the hardest thing for them about caring for their child, 380 (44.8%) indicated the demands of physical care; 313 (36.9%) mentioned emotional factors (such as grieving, remorse, and concerns about personal care); 73 (8.6%) indicated psychological factors (such as interactions with spouse, family, community, loneliness, isolation, and social networks). Lack of privacy was the category label given for the feelings of intrusion that 26 (3.1%) caregivers experienced because of professionals coming into their home to offer services. Twelve responses

(1.4%) were categorized as other, and 44 caregivers (5.2%) indicated nothing was especially hard or did not respond.

In response to the question, "What is the best thing for the caregiver about caring for the child at home?" The most frequent answers were the opportunity for the child to share time ($n = 221$, 26.1%), the opportunity to demonstrate love for the child ($n = 207$, 24.4%), and integration of the child into the family ($n = 184$, 21.7%). It is interesting to note that only three caregivers indicated nothing or gave no response for this question. Caregivers were eager to share what it meant to have the child in the home.

The two most important assets caregivers thought parents should have were information and personal strength. Information refers to knowledge about caring for the child, community resources, and the ability to recognize what is normal development in the child. Personal strength refers to the stamina needed to provide physical care to the child day after day and often in isolation. Two hundred sixty-four caregivers (31.1%) specified knowledge about caring for the child, 58 (6.8%) specified community resources, and 74 (8.7%) specified recognition of normal development. The second most important factor included psychosocial concerns. Two hundred thirty-eight caregivers (28.1%) noted personal strength, 122 (14.4%) specified emotional responsibility, 23 (2.7%) specified social support, and 36 (4.2%) specified advocacy.

Discussion

The majority of primary caregivers were the children's mothers, who were typically educated, middle-class women. The majority of families resided in urban/suburban areas and were intact—that is husband, wife, and children resided together. Mothers typically assumed the role of caregiver for the children. There is no evidence that religion was a significance variable in the study. The level of education and economic level may be important factors in how participants responded. Most were verbal, eager to share, and able to describe their experiences of caring for the child in the home. The supportive device-dependent (SDD) group had the largest number of siblings living in the home.

Of those caregivers who indicated they received help from someone other than a professional, most received it from relatives. It appears that others who helped provided primarily respite care. It is interesting to note that for the ventilator-dependent group ($n = 91$) only 41 caregivers received help from others (relatives, friends, neighbors, sitters, etc.). It is likely that the caregivers of ventilator-dependent children had more help from professionals or carried the burden themselves.

Most of the caregivers did not work outside of the home, but 60% of those who did work outside of their home noted that a member of the family had to take off from work to take their technology-dependent children to hospital or clinic appointments. Most of the caregivers who worked outside the home did so on a part-time basis. Most of the families owned a car or a truck and had insurance or Medicaid benefits. Finances were influenced but did not appear to be the major burden, as demonstrated in an earlier study (Fleming et al., 1994). Based on caregiver responses, the hardest aspects for over 300 of them were providing physical care for the children and handling emotional concerns. It is interesting to note that only 56% of the caregivers indicated they were pleased with the way the nurse cared for their child. This may account for the more than 80% of caregivers indicating a need for information about care.

Caregivers indicated personal strength and knowledge about care as the two most important assets a parent should have in providing care in the home for these children. Their responses reflected that the need for information about physical care and community resources. Their responses indicated, too, that they had psychosocial concerns. More information is needed about family-centered home care, specifically about how families adapt to and cope with the burden of caring for technology-dependent children in the home. Although much care was taken to ensure a representative sample, a smaller percentage of African American (10%), Hispanic (4.5%), and Asian (1.4%) families participated. It appears that these families and lower-income white families may not be using public or private home health care agencies to the same extent that middle- and upper-income white families are using them to assist in the care of children and youth who are dependent on technological devices in the home. Because minority populations are increasing, more information may be needed to determine whether technology-dependent minority children, particularly Hispanic and African American children, are being cared for in the home and what characteristics they have.

A major limitation of this study is that data were collected from telephone interviews, limiting the ability to validate the accuracy of all of the information obtained. Another limitation is that some Hispanic (fewer than 15) caregivers could not participate because the investigators did not have a Spanish interview guide. There also is the possibility that some families without phones did not volunteer in spite of a plan procedure to handle participants without phones. All respondents who participated had access to a telephone.

Implications

There are two policy and practice implications of this study that are important. The more significant implication is that caregivers believe what is needed more than anything else is knowledge about how to care for their technology-dependent children. Professionals who make up the discharge planning team have a responsibility to ensure that caregivers receive adequate information about the care of the child before discharge. The team leader and coordinator of the discharge planning team have a unique responsibility to ensure that appropriate planning for care in the home is done with team members before the child is discharged. Including the home care nurse in the discharge planning conference is desirable to aid in facilitating the continuity of care. Professionals who provide care in the home also need to ensure that the caregiver has appropriate information as changes occur in the developmental and health status of the child. It is important that they are sensitive to the needs of the family and aid the family in meeting its needs effectively and in an efficient manner. Teaching families by providing information and demonstrations to meet needs such as formula care, tracheotomy care, changing and caring for feeding tubes, intravenous care, signs and symptoms of respiratory distress, infection, neurological impairments, feeding intolerance, and IV infiltration are but a few of the needs families have identified. The public health or visiting nurses most often are the constant in the family's life. They may need special training, too, to prepare for providing in the home the technical care that may be required.

The second implication is that the primary diagnosis and the OTA (1987) classification may not be adequate to describe some of these children. One finding showed many of the children in the OTA-defined categories had additional problems. This finding has important implications for recognizing that the OTA categories are useful, but that combining categories may be appropriate for some children who are technology dependent. Recognizing this factor may be useful in enhancing assessment of these children's dependency needs.

SUMMARY

The characteristics presented in this chapter provide some information about the caregivers of children and youth who are technology dependent and their families. Some of the information is general. The impact on the family can be overwhelming.

Respite care seems important in helping these families cope. "Respite care is not a frill. It is a necessity. It is something all families need and deserve. The necessity for respite care must be communicated to those in charge of creating and funding new programs at the federal and state levels" (Association for Care of Children's Health, 1984, p. 52). The theory of dependent care has tremendous potential for use in research of families that provide the caregiver role for children who are technology dependent and cared for in the home. Taylor, Renpenning, Neuman, and Hart (2001) indicated that there are still elements of theory that need further development, such as specifying the enabling abilities of the dependent care agency and verifying and formalizing its various elements. The focus for researchers, educators, and health care practitioners must be on the individual children in the families as well as the parents. Challenges and opportunities face health care providers as they provide care to this growing population of children, youth, and their families.

REFERENCES

Association for Care of Children's Health. (1984). Approaches to respite care. P. M. Smith Facilitator in *Home Care for Children with Serious Handicapping Conditions.* A report of a conference held in Houston, Texas.

Baldwin-Meyers, A. A., & Oppenheimer, E. A. (1996). Quality of life and quality of care data from 7 year pilot for home ventilator patients. *Journal of Ambulatory Care Management, 19*(1), 46–59.

Bandura, A. (1977). Self-efficacy: Toward a unifying theory of behavioral change. *Psychology Review, 9,* 191–215.

Barth, R. R., Blythe, B. J., Schinke, S. P., & Shilling, R. R. (1983). Self-control training with maltreating parents. *Child Welfare, 62,* 313–324.

Beresford, B. (1996). Coping with the care of a severely disabled child. *Health and Social Care in the Community, 4*(1), 30–40.

Bronfenbrenner, V. (1977). Toward an experimental ecology of human development. *American Psychologist, 32,* 513–531.

Campbell, T. (1998). Caring for the technology-dependent child: A case study. *NURS Prax N.2., 13*(2), 5–10.

Carlsson, G., Hakansson, A., Rubensson, A., & Finkel, Y. (1997). Home parenteral nutrition (HPN) in children in Sweden. *Pediatric Nursing, 23*(3), 272–274.

Cassel, J. (1974). Psychosocial processes and stress: Theoretical formulations. *International Journal of Health Services, 4,* 471–482.

Chinn, P. L. (1974). *Child health maintenance.* St. Louis, MO: C. V. Mosby.

Cobb, S. (1976). Social support as a moderator of life stress. *Psychosomatic Medicine, 38,* 300–314.

Cohen, M. H. (1999). The technology-dependent child and the socially marginalized family: A provisional framework. *Qualitative Health Research, 9*(5), 654–668.

Crinic, K. A., Fredrich, W. N., & Greenberg, M. T. (1983). Adaptation of families with mentally retarded children: A model of stress, coping and family ecology. *American Journal of Mental Deficiency, 88,* 125–138.

Dimagio, G., & Sheetz, A. (1983). The concerns of mothers caring for an infant on an apnea monitor. *MCH: The American Journal of Maternal Child Nursing, 8,* 294–297.

Duvall, E. M. (1971). *Family development.* Philadelphia: J. B. Lippincott.

Duvall, E. M. (1977). *Marriage and family development.* Philadelphia: J. B. Lippincott.

Feetham, S. (1984). Family research: Issues and directions for nursing. In H. H. Werley & J. J. Fitzpatrick (Eds.), *Annual review of nursing research, Vol. V* (pp. 3–26). New York: Springer.

Feinberg, E. (1999). Enlarging the paradigm: A public-private partnership in the design of a service plan for a young child with special health care needs. *Infants and Young Children, 11*(4), 97–96.

Fleming, J. (1985). Maternal-child nursing in the decade ahead. *American Journal of Maternal-Child Nursing, 10*(6), 369–370, 374, 376.

Fleming, J. (1996). *Characteristics of high-tech home care of technology-dependent children.* Unpublished report, University of Kentucky, Lexington.

Fleming, J., Challela, M., Eland, J., Hornick, R., Johnson, P., Martinson, I., Nativo, D., Nokes, K., Riddle, I., Steele, N., Sudela, K., Thomas, R., Turner, Q., Yoshioka, B., & Young, A. (1994). Impact on the family of children who are technology dependent and cared for in the home. *Pediatric Nursing, 20*(4), 379–388.

Garbarino, J. (1983). What do we know about child maltreatment? *Children and Youth Services Review, 5,* 3–6.

Haddad, A. M. (1996). The evolution of high-tech home care. In L. A. Garski (Ed.), *High Tech Home Care Manual.* Gaithersburg, MD: Aspen.

Hammer, J. (2000). Home ventilation in children: Indications and practical aspects. *Schweizerische-Medizinische-Wechenscrift, 130*(49), 1894–1902.

Hill, R., & Hansen, D. (1960). The identification of conceptual frameworks utilized in family study. *Marriage and Family Living, 22,* 308.

Hill, R., & Hansen, D. (1964). Families under stress. In H. T. Christensen (Ed.), *Handbook of marriage and family* (pp. 712–819). Chicago: Rand McNally.

Hobbs, N., Perrin, J. M., & Ireys, H. T. (1993). *Chronically ill children and their families.* San Francisco: Jossey-Bass.

Kantor, D., & Lehr, W. (1975). *Inside the family.* New York: Harper & Row.

Kiernan, B. (1995). Parents' perception of family functioning and parental coping in families of chronically ill children dependent upon home intervention therapy. Doctoral dissertation, University of Kentucky, Lexington.

Knoll, J. (1992). Being a family: The experience of raising a child with a disability or chronic illness. *American Association Mental Retardation, 18,* 167–174.

Lazarus, R. S. (1977). *Psychological stress and coping process.* New York: McGraw-Hill.

Lazarus, R. S., & Folkman, S. (1984). *Stress, appraisal and coping.* New York: Springer.

Lynn, D. B. (1974). *The father! His role in child development.* Monterey, CA: Wadsworth.

MacElveen-Hoehn, P., & Eyres, S. (1984). Social support and vulnerability: State of art in relation to families and children. In B. Raff, K. Barnard, & P. Brandt (Eds.), *Social support and families of vulnerable infants.* New York: March of Dimes Birth Defects Foundation, Vol. 20.

Martinson, I. (1976). *Home care for the dying child.* New York: Appleton Century Crofts.

Maurano, L. W. (1994). Community and home care. In C. L. Betz, M. Hunsberger, & S. Wright (Eds.), *Family-centered nursing care of children* (2nd ed., pp. 782–804). Philadelphia: W. B. Saunders.

McCaleb, A., & Luther, I. S. (1996). Characteristics and coping patterns of families with infants on home apnea monitoring. *Issues in Comprehensive Pediatric Nursing,* 19(2), 81–92.

McCubbin, M. A. (1989). Family stress and family strengths: A comparison of single and two-parent families with handicapped children. *Research in Nursing and Health,* 12, 101–110.

McGarth, J. (1970). *Social and psychological factors in stress.* New York: Holt, Rinehart and Winston.

Miles, M., Holditch-Davis, D., Burchinal, P., & Nelson, D. (1999). Distress and growth outcomes of mothers of medically fragile infants. *Nursing Research,* 48(3), 129–140.

Moldow, D., Armstrong, D., Henry, W., & Martinson, I. (1982). The cost of home care for dying children. *Medical Care,* 20, 1154–1160.

O'Brien, M. E. (2001). Living in a house of cards: Family experience long-term childhood technology dependence. *Journal of Pediatric Nursing,* 16(1), 13–22.

Office of Technology Assessment of the Congress of the United States. (1986). Personal communication.

Office of Technology Assessment of the Congress of the United States (1987). Technology-dependent children: Hospital vs. home care. Washington, DC: U.S. Government Printing Office.

Otto, H. A. (1963). A framework for assessing family strengths. In A. M. Reinhardt & M. D. Quinn (Eds.), *Family-centered community nursing: A socio-cultural framework* (p. 88). St. Louis, MO: C. V. Mosby.

Pless, I. B. (1974). Theoretical and practical consideration in the measurement of outcome. In Gilman, D. G., & Pless, I. B. (Eds.), *Chronic Childhood Illness: Assessment of Outcome. A Conference sponsored by the John E. Forgarty International Center for Advanced Study in the Health Sciences and the National Institutes of Health.* Bethesda, MD: U.S. Department of Health, Education and Welfare.

Pless, I. B., & Satterswhite, B. (1973). A measure of family functioning and its application. *Social Science and Medicine,* 7, 613–621.

Quint, R. D., Chesterman, E., Crain, L. S., Winkleby, M., & Boyce, W. T. (1990). Home care of ventilator dependent children: Psychosocial impact on the family. *American Journal of Diseases of Children,* 144(11), 1238–1241.

Rapport, T., & Rosow, I. (1996). An approach to family relationships and role performance in role theory: Concepts and research. In B. Biddle & E. Thomas (Eds.), *Role theory: Concepts and research* (pp. 231–236). New York: Wiley.

Reed, P. G. (1991). Toward a nursing theory of self-transcendence deductive reformation using developmental theories. *Advances in Nursing Science,* 13(4), 64–77.

Reed, S. B. (1991). *Potential for alterations in family process: When a family has a child with cystic fibrosis. International Disability Studies,* 13(4), 146–149.

Scott, D., Oberst, M., & Dropkin, M. (1980). A stress coping model. *Advances in Nursing Science,* 3, 9–23.

Siegel, K., Raveis, V. H., Houts, P., & Mor, V. (1991). Caregiver burden and unmet patient needs. *Cancer, 68*(5), 131–140.

Somerville, R. M. (1972). *Introduction to family life and sex education.* Englewood Cliffs, NJ: Prentice-Hall.

Stein, R. E. K., & Reissman, C. (1980). The development of an impact on family scale: Preliminary findings. *Medical Care, 18*, 465–471.

Taylor, S. G., Renpenning, K. E., Neuman, B. M., & Hart, M. A. (2001). A theory of dependent care: A corollary theory to Orem's Theory of Self-Care. *Nursing Science Quarterly, 14*(1), 39–47.

Tebbi, C. K. (1993). Treatment compliance in childhood and adolescence. *Cancer, 7*(10), 3441–3449.

Thorne, S. E., Radford, M. A., & Armstrong, E. (1977). Gastrostomy in children: Caregiving coping. *Gastroenterology Nursing, 20*(2), 46–53.

Vandvik, I. H., & Eckblad, G. (1991). Mothers of children with recent onset of rheumatic disease. *Journal of Development Behavior Pediatrics, 12*(2), 84–91.

Vogel, T. C., & McSkimming, S. A. (1983). Teaching parents to give indwelling c. v. catheter care. *Nursing, 1*, 55–56.

Watson, J. (1979). *Nursing: The philosophy and science of caring.* Boston: Little, Brown.

Winch, R. F. (1952). *The modern family.* New York: Holt, Rinehart and Winston.

Zajonc, R. B. (1976). Family configuration and intelligence. *Science, 192*(4236), 227–236.

Chapter 7

Stresses and Rewards: The Mental Health Issues of Caregivers

Caring is a difficult concept to translate into measurable terms. It can be viewed as an interactive process between the health care providers and the children who are technology dependent and their families that actualizes growth. Watson (1979) identifies several elements of care. Among them are acceptance of the expression of positive and negative feelings, nonverbal warmth, genuineness, and empathy. Some of the elements seem important to providing support to families with technology-dependent children and youth who are being cared for in the home. Social support, stress, and coping are factors that are likely to affect the mental health of the family caregiver.

STRESS AND COPING:
THE IMPORTANCE OF SOCIAL SUPPORT

The relationship of social support and health status has rapidly developed from a scientific perspective. There is a claim that social support can serve as a buffer to people's responses to stressors. Cassel (1974) and Cobb (1976) point out that under conditions of high life change or chronic exposure to stressors, social support buffers the individual from potentially adverse effects on mood and functioning and facilitates coping and adaptation. Social support is not easily defined or measured because much of it has to do with what the individual perceives. Gender and ethnicity may be associated with perceived supportive strategies. Culturally diverse responses, in terms of supportive strategies that enhance outcomes of personal or family development, also need to be studied.

MacElveen, Hoehn, and Eyres (1984) note six broad categories that tend to be included in most descriptions of social support: emotional concerns, information, appraisal, instrumental aid, social integration, and social participation. Each of the categories covers a variety of concerns.

The dynamics of adaptation are focused on the counterpart to stress, which is coping. There is extensive literature relative to stress and coping behaviors. Much of the of the stress and coping literature is relevant for nursing's contribution to caring and for technology-dependent children receiving care in the home (Bandura, 1977; Lazarus, 1977; Lazarus & Folkman, 1984; McGarth, 1970; Scott, Oberst, & Dropkin, 1980).

Studies done on mechanisms of social support for families with children who have special needs confirm that social support for families is important (Sabbeth & Leventhal, 1984). The presence of adequate support may result in improved family coping. Cenic, Greenberg, Ragozin, Robinson, and Basham (1983) examined the relationships of stress and social support to maternal attitudes. In reviewing behavioral science studies about social support and social network, a number of articles have been published from 1967 to the present. Content domains include general psychosocial, life events, stress and coping, preventive health behaviors, community, and family support. Emphasizing the importance of studying social support in families of home care of children who are technology dependent may provide additional information about this vulnerable population group. Longitudinal studies, which include the culturally diverse populations in society, are needed.

CAREGIVERS

Fleming (1993) found that 457 (53.9%) of 848 caregivers she studied were visited by nursing personnel (e.g., RN, LPN/LVN, aide). Four hundred seven indicated that they were pleased with the way the nurse cared for their child; others indicated they were pleased some of the time, or did not provide a response. It is interesting to note that only 124 (14.6%) indicated they had the resource of respite services; 724 (85.4%) caregivers that were caring for their technology-dependent children in their home did not have respite services. Forty-six (5.4%) indicated they had sitter services, while 802 (94.6%) responded "no" when asked if they had sitter services. Twenty-four (2.8%) had home schooling while 824 (97.2%) responded "no" to home schooling. Keep in mind that the children primarily were from 1 month through 19 years of age, and they functioned at levels much lower than their stated ages. The interpretation of this response and the one that follows about preschool need to be considered in the context noted here. Forty-one (4.8%) used the resource of preschool for their child; 807 (95.2%) did not use this resource. None used hospice care. Six hundred twenty-six (73.8%) of the 848 caregivers indicated they used medical supplies and/or medications in the home.

PSYCHO-EMOTIONAL EFFECTS OF CAREGIVING

The psycho-emotional effects on caregivers and their children who depend on technology to sustain vital body functions is a reality. Those working with children who are technology dependent and their families must face this reality and help them handle these effects and cope with them. Robinson (1997) notes that the majority of caregivers are women. Caregiver burden is experienced by many of those families who care for technology-dependent children in their homes.

Depression, burden, and parental stress have been documented in families who are caregivers (Bull, 2001; Feinberg, 1985; Johnson, 1987). Family caregivers may feel loss of privacy, loneliness, feelings of powerlessness, and loss of control as a result of health care providers coming into their homes (Johnson, 1987; Thompson, Zeman, Fanurik, & Sirotkin-Roses, 1992). If the child needs care that results in increased health care expenditures, it may affect expenditures for health care of other members of the family (Altman, Cooper, & Cunningham, 1999). All of these factors are likely to have some affect on the mental well-being of the family caregiver, particularly the mother who often assumes this role.

IDENTIFICATION OF MENTAL HEALTH PROBLEMS

Further, the mental health of parents with children who are technology dependent may be affected because of the complexity of care, the added stress associated with this complexity, and the feelings that they may have failed in some way. When people perceive themselves as failing, they may think less of themselves and be angry. Their adaptive abilities may become diminished, and they may resort to more primitive mechanisms to try to restore a sense of security and adjustment. They may withdraw from others or deny depressive feelings or that anything has changed, or they may project anger onto others, conveying that others are angry with them. They may develop physical symptoms (somatization) or respond with global anxiety, expressing it openly and to anyone, as a young child does. Sarcasm, blaming, or criticism may be directed at others, especially when those others consider behavior that is being displayed as inappropriate (Murray & Huelskoetter, 1991).

Helping the caregiver maintain a healthy mental health state is paramount. If the caregiver, who typically is the mother, is having mental health difficulties, the entire family is likely to be affected. The parent who is having difficulty with mental health will no doubt be unable to meet the physiological and emotional needs of the child. It is important that the child who is technology dependent not be in a depressed state over time. In order for the child to develop and master tasks to protect himself or herself from depression, the child must have help, attention, and support from the parents. Having a family with a history of mental health problems is a risk factor for childhood problems. The stress and burden that occurs in families caring for technology-dependent children in the home is likely to develop into a problem if the family is unable to cope with caring for the child.

Clinical Assessment

Recognition of a potential parental mental health problem is an important first step as it provides an opportunity for the professional worker to consider ways to intervene and assist the parent. The following may be indicative of signs of a mental health problem:

- Appearance: personal hygiene may be below that expected (hair not groomed, clothes disheveled).
- Verbal response: slow, halting.
- Physical symptoms: hypochondriacal somatic delusions, morbid preoccupation with health.
- Masked symptoms: headache, earache.
- Behavior: memory may not be good for remote or recent events; may be agitated.
- Feeling: may feel sad, distress of the human spirit.

To obtain more definitive information, the following techniques have been used to obtain data needed to help make a nursing diagnosis and to develop a plan of care.

Caregivers and their children sometimes have difficulty expressing themselves and explaining exactly what they are feeling. Using projective techniques allows the parent caregiver and the child to respond indirectly and allows for them to provide multiple responses. Bellack and Fleming (1996) note that unlike objective instruments, projective approaches such as drawings do not limit the number or variety of responses because they are less structured. There are no right or wrong answers, and the caregiver and the child are free to respond without fear. Further, projective techniques, such as associative techniques (when a person is presented with a stimulus, such as the Thermatic Apperception Test for a response), constructive techniques (when a person is required to develop some form of an organized response, such as storytelling or sentence completion), expressive techniques (when the person engages in drawing, painting, or dramatizing) and ordering techniques (which require the person to place items, such as a series of pictures in a desired order) are also relatively free of cultural bias, making it possible to obtain information from the children and their caregiver parents regardless of their age, gender, socioeconomic status, or ethnicity.

The expressive technique of drawing (such as "draw a person" and "kinetic family" drawings) has been successfully used in obtaining data from children and their families. Drawings have been found to be of value in assessing a child or family member's perceptions of stressful or potentially stressful situations. Drawings have been used to aid in understanding children's health conditions (Fleming, 1973). In two studies, drawings were used to gain better understanding of children and their families (Fleming, Holmes, Barton, & Osbahr, 1993; Fleming, Holmes, & Stephens, 1988). The reliability and validity of drawing have been questioned as a technique for obtaining information from persons. Poster (1989) notes that validity of interpreting or scoring children's drawings can be enhanced when someone other than the investigator or test administrator analyzes the results. Drawings could be used as one approach to obtaining data about the emotions of family members—the technology-dependent child, the caregiver parents, and siblings of the child. It can be a nonthreatening, relaxing means of getting the family to do something together. Using colored crayons for drawings might also be revealing.

A direct approach to obtaining information in addressing depressive symptoms in children and their adult caregivers is to use a tool like the Beck Depression Scale. It has a self-rating scale for children and adults that includes suicide. The scale rates depression and can be used to track changes in depression.

The Center for Epidemiologic Studies Depression (CES-D) Scale (Radloff, 1977) has proven to be an effective and valid tool. (See Figure 7.1 for the Questions.) The instrument has been used to assess psychiatric populations, including depressed and nondepressed groups of patients. The scale was developed to be appropriate for use in studies of the epidemiology of depressive symptomatology in the general population. It was intended and expected to identify not only the presence but also the severity of depressive symptomatology. The scale is designed to reflect the current state and to be responsive to changes in state, according to Radloff and Locke (1986). They note that each response is scored from 0 to 3 on a scale of frequency occurring during the last week. The scoring of positive items is reversed, with less frequent occurrences scoring higher. The possible range of scores is 0 to 60, with the higher scores indicating the presence of more symptomatology. Other assessments that are warranted would, of course, be appropriate for the health professional to carry out so that an effective plan of care can be developed for the individual family and child.

Nursing the potentially depressed or depressed family members and/or child who is technology dependent requires the recognition that a mental health problem is present. Individual therapy for the affected person should be provided. The nurse should seek out professional experts such as counselors, psychologists, and psychiatrists to provide the care needed or to guide him/her in delivering the appropriate care.

Leahey's and Wright's (1987) discussion of families and psychosocial problems might serve as a reference source for providing worthwhile information to nurses who are working with families with children who are technology dependent. Families that have psychosocial problems will not function well without intervention. Family therapy becomes the treatment of choice when individual therapy fails. If one family member's improved functioning causes another member's dysfunction, family therapy may be in order. Not all disturbed families, however, will necessarily benefit from therapy that involves all family members.

Bull (2001) notes that coping and social support have been identified as potential mediators of burden. In reviewing 14 studies on interventions for family caregivers, Bull indicates that the majority of studies found no significant differences between the intervention and control groups on depression, burden, and parental stress. The studies reviewed included the use of longitudinal designs, random assignment to intervention, and control groups. Bull's findings regarding depression are supported by Given and Given (1991), who found that for caregivers of the elderly, depression is found regardless of income, the medical diagnosis of the patient, and the

Instructions for Questions: Below is a list of the ways you might have felt or behaved. Please tell me how often you have felt this way during the past week.

Rarely or none of the time (less than 1 day)

Some or a little of the time (1–2 days)

Occasionally or a moderate amount of the time (3–4 days)

Most or all of the time (5–7 days)

During the past week:

I was bothered by things that usually don't bother me.

I did not feel like eating; my appetite was poor.

I felt that I could not shake off the blues even with help from my family or friends.

I felt that I was just as good as other people.

I had trouble keeping my mind on what I was doing.

I felt depressed.

I felt that everything I did was an effort.

I felt hopeful about the future.

I thought my life had been a failure.

I felt fearful.

My sleep was restless.

I was happy.

I talked less than usual.

I felt lonely.

People were unfriendly.

I enjoyed life.

I had crying spells.

I felt sad.

I felt that people dislike me.

I could not get "going."

FIGURE 7.1   CES-D Scale.

length of time care giving has been provided. The expectation then is to minimize depression so that untoward effects do not result for the caregiver, the family, or the child who is technology dependent. Based on their observations and relationship with the family, nurses can provide support as needed as well as identify and refer the family to other professionals, such as a social worker, psychologist, or psychiatrist based on his/her assessment.

Kiernan (1995) found that various dimensions of parental coping included age, income, marital status, and family functioning. She concludes that these factors may be useful in providing optimum ongoing care and support services to families. Adults with a more highly developed sense of spiritual well-being may be less lonely and view life more positively. How a parental caregiver responds may depend on the child's condition, which may range from mild to severe. The more limiting the condition is, the greater the likelihood that the family will not cope well with the situation without a high level of support and knowledge about how to care for the child. When a parent has a child who requires technology for physiological functioning, he or she may go through a coping sequence. It is a reaction to change and may be great enough to produce stress in response to a trauma. The coping, like the grief stages, may be (1) shock and denial, (2) anxiety, (3) anger and/or guilt, and (4) depression. If this premise is correct, the expectation is that parents of children who are technology dependent will at some point be depressed before they are able to cope with the situation of having a child who is technology dependent.

The health care professional needs to use skills of assessment and observation sources such as psychologists and psychiatrists to help plan effective means to help the family caregivers help themselves. Families that are able to work together and that adapt and cope effectively increase family cohesiveness, according to Hiett (1985). The use of informal sources such as family members, neighbors, and other parents of children with disabilities, and formal sources in the community, such as health care facilities, respite centers, and social service agencies, is important for the family if it is to manage the situation and maintain satisfactory mental health. Families of "normal" children have stresses and generally handle them. Evidence suggests that the families of technology-dependent children also will be able to do so if the stress is mediated. Health professionals can help families develop strategies that will be positive reinforcers. The negative associations with disability and the negative physical, psycho-emotional, and psychosocial effects can be abated with assistance from health professionals, particularly nurses who are concerned with holistic care.

The American Nurses Association (2000) considers standards for community-based care, which includes care delivered in partnership with patients in their homes and other areas. The standards cover (1) assessment, (2) diagnosis, (3) outcome identification, (4) planning, (5) implementation (counseling, milieu therapy, promotion of self-care activities, psychobiological interventions, health teaching, case management, health promotion, and health maintenance), and (6) evaluation. Measurement criteria are delineated for each standard. Nurses who work with families who have technology-dependent children are urged to use these standards as needed in caring for those who exhibit mental health difficulties.

Preventing mental health problems in caregiving families of children who are technology dependent and cared for in their homes is preferable to having to treat problems when they become more serious. Technology-dependent children typically may already require multiple services. Coordinating mental health services, if they cannot be provided by the primary care professional who is working with and caring for the family, may be an added stressor for the family. While this chapter offers suggestions for managing and providing the mental health care, it is essential that health care professionals recognize that the effectiveness of such interventions is limited in terms of wide use with children who are technology dependent and their families in the home. Although the approaches have been effective with individual families and their children, there is no definitive base of evidence. Consequently, the approaches proposed are suggested as an initial means for those children who are technology dependent and receiving home care and their families.

REWARDS OF CAREGIVING

Satisfaction may be one of the rewards caregiving parents can experience. Pasley, Gecas, and March (1984) examined stresses and satisfaction of parenting. They found the role of parent is seen as a difficult and complex one, and that the presence of children affects marital satisfaction. These authors found adolescence to be the most difficult stage of parenting, using a sample of fathers ($N = 136$) and mothers ($N = 149$) who responded to a questionnaire dealing with perceptions of parenthood with regard to perceived satisfactions and difficulties for various stages of the family cycle. Younger children (0 to 5 years) were selected by both fathers and mothers as in the best stage. This age group was seen as enjoyable.

In a study of parental satisfaction of 454 families, Chillman (1980) found that both mothers and fathers viewed parenthood as the most important aspect of their family life. The majority of mothers found parenthood more satisfying than their outside employment. Inasmuch as parents, for the most part, are the caregivers of children who are technology dependent and cared for in the home, satisfaction of the caregivers was seen as important in terms of its implications for care of this population.

Factors that have been suggested in the literature that may affect parents, particularly the mother's perception of satisfaction with her child, include the child's behavior (Green, Forehand, & McMahon, 1979), stresses of life (Dohrenwend & Dohrenwend, 1981), marital satisfaction (Hetherington & Parker, 1979), and depression. Furey and Forehand (1984) examined the relationship of seven factors (child behavior, maternal depression, marital satisfaction, extrafamilial interaction, time with child, exercise, and life stresses) to maternal satisfaction. They found that maternal satisfaction in the group of 48 middle-class white mothers studied was high. Using multiple aggression analysis to determine the impact of the predictor variables on maternal satisfaction, they found three primary dimensions that contribute to maternal satisfaction. They were child behavior, maternal depression, and maternal independent activity as measured by exercise. They note that future research should expand the characteristics (e.g., race, social economic status, satisfaction with child) of the sample used in this study. This particular study provides a basis of the factors that perhaps should be considered in determining satisfaction of caregivers who care for children who are technology dependent in the home. Lessing, Swift, Metcalf, and Baum (1992) found that more than 90% of parents were satisfied with the preparation they received before the discharge of their child newly diagnosed with diabetes. The diabetes nurse specialist was seen as the most supportive person in the first year after diagnosis. The greatest source of dissatisfaction was the liaison with schools.

In her study of families of children dependent upon home IV therapy, Kiernan (1995) notes that despite added stress, respondents in this sample were more satisfied with family life and well-being than in the normative sample. Satisfaction may come from knowing that caring for one's child has positive benefits (Teague et al., 1993) and that one is in a supportive relationship. Parents in Kiernan's study also reported higher family cohesion scores than the normative sample.

Of the 848 parent/guardian caregivers of children who were technology dependent and being cared for in the home interviewed by Fleming (1993), 268 (31.6%) noted that they were more satisfied and 302 (35.6%) noted they were as satisfied with the home care their child was receiving as when the child was hospitalized. One hundred forty (16.5%) were less satisfied. One response was missing and 137 either did not know or were not applicable. The preparation the parental caregiver received before bringing the child home was viewed as more than adequate by 236 (27.8%) and adequate by 411 (48.5%) of the 848 caregivers interviewed. One hundred fifteen (13.6%) caregivers felt the preparation was less than adequate, and 71 (8.4%) felt it was not adequate. The other 15 did not know or indicated not applicable. Tables 7.1 through 7.13 indicate areas of satisfaction that Fleming (1993) found from the responses of caregivers to the Personal Resource Questionnaire (PRQ).

Caregivers responded to questions as to what they felt in terms of satisfaction regarding support from their families and the satisfaction they had from the perspective of caring for their child, having enough finances to provide adequate care, having the opportunity to talk with others about the child, the availability of things they needed to care for the child, the quality of their life in general, the availability of health providers, and the amount of information they had to provide care.

Fleming et al. (1994) note that satisfaction with the quality of the caregiver's life varied significantly among the four types of technology dependency. No effect was found on the caregiver's level of depression or satisfaction when they were controlled for the type of dependency. A logistic regression model was used to predict the logistic odds of respondents with a CES-D score of 16 or above (indicating signs of depression) and a Family APGAR score above the median (indicating satisfaction). A great deal of satisfaction with having enough finances to provide an adequate level of care for their child was found. The analysis, however, showed that the type of dependency is not a significant predictor of depression nor for three of the measures of satisfaction. It was, however, a predictor for respondents who reported a great deal of satisfaction with their general quality of life. Wegener and Aday (1989) note that families of ventilator-dependent children were satisfied with having them at home.

Chronic illness affects a large number of children each year. Among this group are a number of technology-dependent children who are cared for in their homes. Shaw and Halliday (1992) identify the disruption and disability in the lives of caregivers of chronically ill children. The efforts to treat their children as normally as possible are difficult because of the medical devices that many must use, the continuous monitoring of their care, the various treatments they must receive, and the frequency of visits from health professionals.

The families who care for the children who are on ventilators in the home are under a great deal of stress. Caregiver well-being is a factor that health care providers need to seriously consider. Scharer and Dixon (1989) reported on 10 families of ventilator-dependent children cared for in their homes in terms of medical, social, and financial variables. The children ranged from ages 8 months to 16 years of age. The parents of all the children agreed that caring for the children in the home was beneficial to family relations. The children remained stable or improved physically after discharge to their homes. The downsides of having the children at home were loss of privacy, sleep disruptions, limitations on social life, curtailed sibling activities, and financial hardship, although 5 of the 10 families received some type of public funding. Fleming et al. (1994) found that the study on the impact of the family of children who are technology dependent did not support the assumption that children who are technology dependent regardless of type will be a financial burden on the family.

Satisfaction of families with the health care they receive for their children who are technology dependent in the home is an important dimension of health care delivery. The quality of health care services, which includes freedom from accidental injury during treatment, is seen as a critical step in enhancing quality care. Determining the caregiver's level of satisfaction with the care of the technology-dependent child appears to be a valid means of helping to assess the quality of care.

Parental abilities and attitudes are factors that may influence the quality and effectiveness of home care. "A crucial condition for effective home care is that the family wants the child at home, and that it is willing and able to help care for the child or to accept and support a professional caregiver into the household" (Office of Technology Assessment, 1987). Satisfaction with care, whether the family members provide it or a professional provides it, is a factor in the quality and effectiveness.

Three salient findings from study conducted by Warfield, Krauss, Hauser-Cram, Upshaw, and Shonkoff (1999) are noted:

1. Families face a range of stressors, some of which are independent of having a child with a disability (e.g., death in family of an immediate member, decrease in income, deep debt, marital separation, divorce).
2. There is variability among mothers regarding the stress related to being a parent (social isolation, relations with spouse, sense of competence as a parent).
3. Family multivariate analysis characteristics, such as low family cohesion, lower income, and lower levels of family support, found that family cohesion was a robust and durable predictor of both child-related and parenting stress.

It is important to assess the degree to which each parent feels supported by his or her spouse or partner as well as ascertaining the extent to which she or he is able to make mutually supported decisions about family life and to feel emotionally secure in the family setting. Although there are not definitive studies that have examined the relationship between satisfaction, the stresses that affect family caregivers, and the support received by those who care for technology-dependent children in the home, it seems reasonable to conclude that there may be an effect.

CONCLUSION

Satisfaction with the care that caregivers provide with the help of professionals is a factor in the changing health care environment. Optimum care of children who are technology dependent and cared for in their homes is likely to depend to a great extent on caregiver satisfaction. A positive outcome for the family member and the child who is technology dependent is what is important. To achieve such an outcome, interventions that provide support for the families and changes in interactions where they are needed are essential.

Health care professionals who provide care in the current health care environment must recognize that patients'/clients' rights are given more consideration than in the past. Satisfaction of the consumer is an aspect of helping to determine quality of care. As greater emphasis is placed on patients' rights, determination of their satisfaction with care will become more important in assessing quality of care from the consumers' perspective. Educators, researchers, and health care practitioners will need to work together to help consumers understand the dimension of care.

In the case of children who are being cared for in the home and are technology dependent, the concept of social marketing for health seems worthwhile. It is, according to Rothenberg and Kaplan (1990), an attempt to make desirable health messages congruent with the interests and needs of the target population. The opportunity to explore this concept is a challenge open to those who wish to explore it with the population of families who are caring for children who are technology dependent in the home. Community assessments of families who are providing care for their technology-dependent children would be desirable, as those persons who are faced daily with the issues of caring for their children could provide worthwhile information. Further, it is desirable to have persons who are faced with issues in the community to provide their input. Williams and

Yanoshik (2001) indicate that, conventionally, it has been accepted that an accurate understanding of community views on health topics can come only directly from community members. They note that the need for data has increased by community members. The need for data also has increased for managed care, and the methods for obtaining data from community members remain costly. They conducted a use study to determine whether informed health professionals could accurately and less expensively convey community views on health topics and found that there may be limited situations in which health care workers can adequately convey community views. They conclude that community members have an important role in planning and decision-making regarding their health care.

TABLE 7.1   Factors That Infuence the Quality and Effectiveness of Home Care

Statement	Response	N	%
Caregivers agree on resources, finance, time, and outings	Strongly agree	222	26.2
	Agree	321	37.9
Illness is causing financial problems for the family	Strongly agree	127	26.2
	Agree	306	36.1
Time is lost from work because of hospital appointments	Strongly agree	123	21.6
	Agree	337	39.7
Hours of time worked were cut back to care for child	Strongly agree	183	21.6
	Agree	199	23.5
There isn't much time left over for other family members after child care	Strongly agree	116	13.7
	Agree	332	39.2
The family gives up things because of child's illness	Strongly agree	227	26.8
	Agree	409	48.3
Caregivers have little desire to go out be cause of their child's illness	Strongly agree	75	8.8
	Agree	254	30.0
Sometimes caregivers have to change so- cial plans because of child's illness	Strongly agree	181	21.3
	Agree	452	53.3

TABLE 7.2   Satisfaction with Child Care

Response	N	%
A great deal	704	83.0
Fair amount	119	14.0
Not much	18	2.1
None at all	3	0.4
Do not know	3	0.4
Refused	1	0.1

TABLE 7.3   Satisfaction with Enough Finances to Provide Good Care

Response	N	%
A great deal	409	48.2
Fair amount	281	33.1
Not much	101	11.9
None at all	49	5.8
Not applicable	3	0.4
Do not know	4	0.5
Refused	1	0.1

TABLE 7.4   Opportunity to Talk with Others About My Child

Response	N	%
A great deal	449	52.9
Fair amount	297	35.0
Not much	59	7.0
None at all	33	3.9
Not applicable	3	0.4
Do not know	6	0.7
Refused	1	0.1

TABLE 7.5 Satisfaction in Obtaining Things Needed to Care for My Child

Response	N	%
A great deal	522	61.6
Fair amount	264	31.1
Not much	39	4.6
None at all	18	2.1
Do not know	4	0.5
Refused	1	0.1

TABLE 7.6 Satisfaction with Quality of Life in General

Response	N	%
A great deal	387	45.7
Fair amount	342	40.3
Not much	81	9.6
None at all	34	4.0
Do not know	3	0.4
Refused	1	0.1

TABLE 7.7 Satisfaction with Availability of Health Care Providers

Response	N	%
A great deal	529	62.4
Fair amount	253	29.8
Not much	48	5.7
None at all	15	1.8
Do not know	2	0.2
Refused	1	0.1

TABLE 7.8   Satisfaction with Amount of Information I Have to Provide Care

Response	N	%
A great deal	538	63.4
Fair amount	237	27.9
Not much	50	5.9
None at all	14	1.7
Not applicable	3	0.4
Do not know	5	0.6
Refused	1	0.1

TABLE 7.9   Satisfaction with Family's Response to My Emotions

Response	N	%
Always	377	44.5
Almost always	187	22.1
Some of the time	195	23.0
Hardly ever	46	5.4
Never	40	4.7
Refused	3	0.4

TABLE 7.10   Satisfaction with Family and Time We Share Together

Response	N	%
Always	313	36.9
Almost always	225	26.5
Some of the time	210	24.8
Hardly ever	56	6.6
Never	38	4.5
Not applicable	2	0.2
Do not know	1	0.1
Refused	3	0.4

TABLE 7.11   Satisfaction with Support from Family When Something Is Troubling Me

Response	N	%
Always	447	52.7
Almost always	163	19.2
Some of the time	162	19.1
Hardly ever	36	4.2
Never	36	4.2
Not applicable	1	0.1
Refused	3	0.4

TABLE 7.12   Satisfaction with the Way Family Talks Over or Shares Problems with Me

Response	N	%
Always	348	41.0
Almost always	185	21.8
Some of the time	208	24.5
Hardly ever	60	7.1
Never	42	5.0
Do not know	2	0.2
Refused	3	0.4

TABLE 7.13   Satisfaction with the Family's Acceptance of My Wish for New Activities or Directions

Response	N	%
Always	368	43.4
Almost always	194	22.9
Some of the time	190	22.4
Hardly ever	46	5.4
Never	41	4.8
Not applicable	1	0.1
Do not know	5	0.6
Refused	3	0.4

REFERENCES

Altman, B., Cooper, P., & Cunningham, P. (1999). The case of disability in the family: Impact on health care utilization and expenditures for non-disabled members. *Milbank Quarterly, 77*(1), 39–75.

American Nurses Association. (2000). *Scope and standards of mental health nursing practice.* Washington, DC: American Nurses Publishing.

Bandura, A. (1977). Self-efficacy: Toward unifying theory of behavioral change. *Psychological Review, 9*, 191–215.

Bellack, J., & Fleming, J. (1996). The use of projective techniques in pediatric nursing research from 1984 to 1993. *Journal of Pediatric Nursing, 11*(1), 10–27.

Bull, M. (2001). Interventions for women as family caregivers. In J. J. Fitzpatrick, D. Taylor, & N. F. Woods (Eds.), *Annual review of nursing research, Vol. 9: Women's health research* (pp. 25–42). New York: Springer.

Cassel, J. (1974). Psychological processes and stress: Theoretical formulations. *International Journal of Health Services, 4*, 471–482.

Chillman, C. (1980). Parent satisfactions, concerns and goals for their children. *Family Relations, 29*, 339–345.

Cobb, S. (1976). Social support as a moderator of life stress. *Psychosomatic Medicine, 38*, 300–314.

Dohrenwend, B. S., & Dohrenwend, B. P. (Eds.). (1981). *Stressful life events and their contexts.* New York: Prodist.

Feinberg, E. A. (1985). Family stress in pediatric home care. *Caring, 4*, 38–41.

Fleming, J. (1993). *Home care of technology-dependent children: Satisfaction.* Unpublished report, College of Nursing, University of Kentucky, Lexington.

Fleming, J., Challela, M., Eland, J., Hornick, R., Johnson, R., Martinson, I., Nativio, D., Nokes, K., Riddle, I., Steele, N., Sudela, K., Thomas, R., Turner, Q., Wheeler, B., & Young, A. (1994). Impact on the family of children who are technology dependent and cared for in the home. *Pediatric Nursing, 20*(4), 379–388.

Fleming, J. W. (1973). Children's drawings and research in understanding health conditions. *Nursing Research Reports, 5–7.*

Fleming, J. W., Holmes, S., Barton, L., & Osbahr, B. (1993). Differences in color preferences of well school age children and those in varying stages of illness. *Maternal-child Nursing Journal, 21*, 130–142.

Fleming, J. W., Holmes, S., & Stephens, L. (1988). Color drawings: A means of identifying problems in children. *Journal of National Black Nurses Association, 3*, 36–44.

Furey, W., & Forehand, R. (1984). An examination of predictors of mother's perceptions of satisfaction with their children. *Journal of Social and Clinical Psychology, 2*(3), 230–243.

Given, B., & Given, C. W. (1991). Family care giving for the elderly. In J. J. Fitzpatrick, R. Taunton, & A. Jacox (Eds.), *Annual review of nursing research.* New York: Springer.

Green, K. D., Forehand, R. L., & McMahon, R. J. (1979). Parental manipulation of compliance and noncompliance in normal and deviant children. *Behavior Modification, 3*, 245–266.

Heitt, K. (1985). Fragile children: Ann Marie. *Caring, 4*, 11.

Hetherington, E. M., & Parker, R. D. (1979). *Child psychology: A contemporary point of view* (2nd ed.). New York: McGraw-Hill.

Johnson, D. L. (1987). Possible long-term effects of high technology on the child and family. *Focus on Critical Care, 14*(4), 43–50.

Kiernan, B. (1995). *Parents' perceptions of family functioning and parental coping in families of chronically ill children dependent upon home intravenous therapy.* Doctoral dissertation, University of Kentucky, Lexington.

Lazarus, R. S. (1977). *Psychological stress and coping process.* New York: McGraw-Hill.

Lazarus, R. S., & Folkman, S. (1984). *Stress, appraisal and coping.* New York: Springer.

Leahey, M., & Wright, M. L. (1987). *Families and psychosocial problems.* Springhouse, PA: Springhouse.

Lessing, D. W., Swift, P. G., Metcalf, M. A., & Baum, J. A. (1992). Newly diagnosed diabetes: A study of parental satisfaction. *ARCH Dis. Child, 67*(8), 1011–1013.

Martinson, I. (1976). *Home care for the dying child.* New York: Appleton Century Crofts.

McElveen-Hoehn, P., & Eyres, S. (1984). Social support and vulnerability: State of the art in relation to families and children. In B. Raff, K. Barnard, & P. Brandt (Eds.), *Families of vulnerable infants.* New York: March of Dimes Birth Defects Foundation, Vol. 20.

McGarth, J. (1970). *Social and psychological factors in stress.* New York: Holt, Rinehart and Winston.

Moldow, D., Armstrong, D., Henry, W., & Martinson, I. (1982). The cost of home care for dying children. *Medical Care, 20,* 1154–1160.

Murray, R. B., & Huelskoetter, M. M. (1991). *Psychiatric/mental health nursing giving emotional care.* Norwalk, CT: Appleton & Lange.

Office of Technology Assessment. (1987). Technology-dependent children: Hospital vs. home care—a technical memorandum. Washington, DC: U.S. Government Printing Office.

Pasley, K., Gecas, V., & March, (1984). Stresses and satisfactions of the parental role. *The Personnel and Guidance Journal,* 400–404.

Poster, E. C. (1989). The use of projective assessment techniques in pediatric research. *Journal of Pediatric Nursing, 4,* 26–35.

Radloff, L. (1977). The CES-D Scale: A self-report depression scale for research in general population. *Applied Psychological Measures, 1,* 385–401.

Radloff, L., & Locke, B. (1986). The Community Mental Health Assessment Survey and CES-D Scale. In M. Weissman, J. Myers, & C. Ross (Eds.), *Community surveys of psychiatric disorders series in psychosocial epidemiology, vol. 4.* New Brunswick, NJ: Rutgers University Press.

Robinson, K. M. (1997). Family care giving. Who provides care and at what cost? *Nursing Economics, 15,* 243–247.

Rothenberg, R. B., & Kaplan, J. P. (1990). Chronic disease in the 1990's. *Annual Review of Public Health, 11,* 267–296.

Sabbeth, B., & Leventhal, J. (1984). Marital adjustment to chronic childhood illness: A critique of literature. *Pediatrics, 93,* 762–767.

Scharer, K., & Dixon, D. M. (1989). Managing chronic illness: Parents with a ventilator dependent child. *Journal of Pediatric Nursing, 4,* 236–247.

Scott, D., Oberst, M., & Dropkin, M. (1980). A stress coping model. *Advances in Nursing Science, 3,* 9–23.

Shaw, M. C., & Halliday, P. H. (1992). The family crisis and chronic illness: An evolutionary model. *Journal of Advanced Nursing, 17*(5), 537–543.

Sweeney, R., & Neff, M. (2001). NMHA launches campaign for children's mental health. *American Family Physician, 63*(12), 2319.

Teague, B., Fleming, J., Wolfe, J., Castle, G., Kiernan, B., Lobo, M., & Riggs, I. (1993). "High tech" home care for children with chronic health conditions: A pilot study. *Journal of Pediatric Nursing: Nursing Care of Children and Families, 8*(4), 226–231.

Thompson, R. J., Zeman, J. L., Fanurik, D., & Sirotkin-Roses, M. (1992). The role of parent stress and coping and family functioning in parent and child adjustment in Duchen muscular dystrophy. *Journal of Clinic Psychology, 48*(1), 9–11.

Warfield, M. E., Krauss, M. W., Hauser-Cram, P., Upshur, C. C., & Shonkoff, J. P. (1999). Adaptation during early childhood among mothers of children with disabilities. *Journal of Developmental Behavioral Pediatrics, 20*(1), 9–16.

Watson, J. (1979). *Nursing: The philosophy and science of caring.* Boston: Little, Brown.

Wegener, D., & Aday, L. (1989). Home care for ventilator assisted children: Predicting family stress. *Pediatric Nursing, 15,* 371–376.

Williams, R., & Yanoshik, K. (2001). Can you do a community assessment without talking to the community? *Journal of Community Health, 26*(4), 233.

Chapter 8

Quality Care

Q uality care is not a new concept. It has become a major public issue and was intensified in 1999–2000 as a result of the Institute of Medicine's reports on the extent of errors in health care (IOM, 1999, 2000). The concept of quality care according to Abdellah and Levine (1994) implies adherence to standards that describe the accepted way in which technical and interpersonal activities should be carried out. Quality care has been broadly defined as desirable achievable health care (Wenzel, 1992). Concerns about patient safety and reduction of medical errors have prompted legislators, states, and professional health care organizations to address the issue of quality improvement in the delivery of care.

IOM (1999) and IOM (2000) are examples of a nationally recognized organization demonstrating of a concern for quality care. The Massachusetts Hospital Association (MHA) is an example of a state organization's concern. The MHA is a founding member of a broad-based coalition committed to working in a cooperative spirit to share information about the causes of errors and strategies for prevention. The coalition is dedicated to improving systems to prevent errors and moving from a culture of blame and punishment to a culture of safety. Legislation has been introduced to establish a center in Massachusetts to focus on increasing patient safety and reducing medical errors. The center would be named the Betsy Lehman Center for Patient Safety and Medical Error Reduction, in honor of the late *Boston Globe* health columnist, who died in 1994 (Collier, 2000). The Agency for Health Care Policy and Research, a governmental agency, has released the Health Care Cost and Utilization Project Quality Indicators (HCUPQs) (Agency for Health Care Policy and Research, 1998). This tool covers three dimensions of care: avoidable hospital outcomes, appropriateness of inpatient procedures, and potentially avoidable hospital admissions. The third dimension may be very relevant to children who are dependent on technology and are being cared for in their home. The Agency for Health Care Policy and Research has several databases that may be useful in studying quality care from a perspective of an inpatient who will be discharged to home care.*

RECENT ACTIVITIES

Quality of health care delivered in the United States has become a frontline issue, along with the traditional concerns about costs and access to care. Quality of care was highlighted in a House of Delegates background document presented at the 2000 American Nurses Association (ANA) Convention (Wakefield, Maddox, & Bull, 2000). Considering that nurses make up the largest group of health care professionals in the workforce and that they not only deliver care but also are involved in patient care education and research, it was and is essential that the professional organization of nursing address the issue of quality. Among activities of ANA noted in the document at the convention were

- Nursing-Sensitive Quality Indicators Initiative established through scientific research the connection between nursing interventions, nursing staffing levels, and positive patient outcomes.
- Magnet Nursing Services Recognition Program for Excellence in Nursing Services recognizes excellence in the provision of nursing services and acknowledges those institutions committed to delivery of quality nursing services.
- Principles for Nurse Staffing establishes parameters for examining appropriate staffing levels necessary for the delivery of quality patient care.

This information along with information about ANA's active involvement in the formulation of Healthy People 2010 objectives was provided to delegates at the convention (Wakefield et al., 2000).

Professional standards of care are basic to the consideration of quality of care. To provide quality care, one must ascertain what constitutes quality care and then perform to meet the attributes that constitute quality. The service nurses provide to children who are technology dependent and

---

*Researchers and practitioners interested in more information about the HCUPQs or the databases may access the World Wide Web site *http://www.achcpr.gov* or write to the Director of the Center for Organization and Delivery Studies Agency for Health Care Policy and Research, 2101 East Jefferson Street, Suite 500, Rockville, MD 20852.

their families must represent a means to improve the child's physical and emotional status as quickly as possible, to prevent further disability, to promote the health and well-being of the child and the family, to involve the child and family caregivers with a definitive role in decision making, and to work with other members of the team in facilitating resources the family needs.

Bennett and Tibbitts (1989) discuss the importance of humanizing health care in a technological society, stating, "To block the threat to humanity, in the health care environment, we must be quick to perceive or apprehend the absence of balance in the scientific and human dimensions of work."

Concepts such as total quality management and quality assurance programs are associated with the quality control and the monitoring of quality. What will make a difference in the care of children who are technology dependent and cared for in their home is to develop care that will be deemed as excellent. The challenge for nurses is to conduct research, transmit knowledge, and use in practice those skills that maximize quality performance.

To determine the quality of health services for those receiving home care, there is tremendous need for data, approaches and tools. Outcomes are thought to be a means of determining quality care. The measuring of outcomes, however, may not be an effective approach because of the problems that are presented. According to Abdellah and Levine (1994), the foremost problems are the intervening and confounding variables that intrude on the relationship between interventions and end results. They also note that outcomes may be difficult to define operationally, thus reducing external validity. These authors note that measuring of process and structure presents fewer problems than measuring outcomes. They identify three areas for future developments in the measurement of quality in nursing: (1) assessment methodology, (2) practice guidelines, and (3) quality assurance programs.

Bennett and Tibbitts (1989) delineate the following as means to enhance total quality:

- commitment
- assessment
- networking
- direction
- strategic planning
- organizational change

- prepared leadership
- human resource management
- systemic integration
- participation of employee
- monitoring, evaluation, and improvement
- sustaining and extending

These elements seem important still for health care organizations that provide services for those children receiving home care.

Parent satisfaction is recognized by many health care providers as a legitimate measure of health care quality (Steiber & Krowinski, 1990). Patient satisfaction with health care is important in understanding the functioning of a health care system. From a practice perspective, patient management/care represents the outcome of helping the family have a degree of satisfaction in facilitating the child who is technology dependent toward independence in their activities of daily living.

Following are definitions of nursing outcome perspectives of some nurse scholars/theorists. All of them can reflect quality of care from a perspective of outcomes of care. Smith (1996) indicates that the problems disrupting quality of life that are commonly reported by caregivers who provide technological care include burdens of physical care, financial strain, and difficulty coping with individual role and schedule disruption. Since nursing care is an important dimension in working with families, using any one of the theorists below, or a combination of them, to design intervention or research evaluation projects may be worthwhile in gaining knowledge to minimize the burdens experienced in caring for children who are technology dependent.

Nightingale—Indicates that nursing is a calling and provides comfort and well-being.

Johnson—Nursing provides an external regulatory force to integrate client in maintaining balance; sense of well-being and relief of tension and discomfort with the ultimate goal of internal and interpersonal equilibrium

Peplau—Nursing involves a therapeutic interpersonal process; personality development and maximum productivity and health and wellness

Henderson—Nursing assists individuals in performance of activities that contribute to health or recovery; independence

Orem—Nurses assist individuals in managing systems of therapeutic self-care; it takes into consideration the soundness and wholeness of developed human structures and bodily and mental functioning.

Leininger—Nurses use culturally based actions to assist and/or support a person or group to ameliorate a human condition; they are concerned with individual or group well-being and quality with cultural congruence.

Roy—Nurses promote adaptation; they enhance positive life processes and patterns of functioning.

Watson—Nurses are concerned with human caring; moral and ethical dimensions of care are emphasized; knowledge; self-reverence; self-healing and self-care processes.

Neuman—Nurses reduce stress to affect optimal functioning; stabilize system to optimal wellness; and

Rogers—Nurses facilitate unitary human beings: patterns are manifestations of human experiences.

Neale (2001) notes the importance of understanding nursing's contribution to health care. She does a creditable job of reviewing 18 theoretical perspectives regarding patient outcomes and indicates that the implications for nurses are substantial. This author agrees with her position. Outstanding or excellent performance by health care professionals in caring for this population and working with their families and other members of the team is best captured by something that has been said about the Hallmark Company, which has been called one of the best companies to work for in the United States, "Excellence is an aspiration, an attitude, a pursuit, a working together, aspiring to the fullness of our potential, always in the pursuit of higher standards, determined to do everything we do better." Excellence is found in caring, in trying, in doing, and in working together. Naturally, to perform at a high level, one must have the knowledge and skills to be prepared to perform. The implications for nurses involved in helping families with outcomes that are satisfactory for them and their children are pertinent to the dynamics of the changes evolving in health care and the care of this population group.

Ascertaining the family's level of stress, level of support, and satisfaction with the care of its children is an appropriate means of obtaining information that will help in planning and providing effective care in the home for children who are technology dependent. Health care practitioners may find it helpful to use objective means of determining stress, feelings of support, and feelings of satisfaction in assessing parental caregivers. There are several questions that could be used to help ascertain parental satisfaction (see Figure 8.1). These questions have been of value in talking with parents, mostly mothers of children being assisted with medical technology.

Responses to each question should be "agree" or "disagree."

1. _____ is dependent on technology.
    (name of child)

2. I enjoy being his/her parent.

3. When caring for _____, I would like to be doing
                      (name of child)
    something else.

4. I enjoy taking care of _____.
                            (name of child)

5. I feel burdened with the many demands that are required to care for

    _____.
    (name of child)

6. I interact with _____ as much as I can as it's
                      (name of child)
    important to me that he/she continues to develop in spite of his/her
    health problem(s) that necessitate the use of technology.

7. I would prefer working outside of the home and have professionals
    care for _____.
              (name of child)

8. My husband/wife should have more involvement in caring for

    _____.
    (name of child)

9. _____ care takes a lot of time and is routine
    (name of child)
    and not challenging.

10. _____ care helps bring the family together.
    (name of child)

11. There is so little time for activities other than care of

    _____.
    (name of child)

FIGURE 8.1   Satisfaction with parenthood of child who is technology
dependent.

The questions serve basically as a screening tool to learn more about how parental caregivers feel about their caregiving role.

Illness in a child serves as both an outcome to be moderated as well as a stressor to the family (Wamboldt & Wamboldt, 2000). Both the child and members of the family must be considered in terms of their coping and satisfaction with their lives. Consultation with a child and adolescent psychiatrist may help practitioners improve the way a family manages a child's illness. The psychiatrist may help in the treatment of psychological symptoms in the ill child or family member. The child's illness and technology dependency may have an effect on the entire family, as well as different effects on each member. Decreasing family problems and concerns may help the family have a higher level of satisfaction in caring for the child who is technology dependent and, consequently, result in increased quality of care and effectiveness. When serving as a consultant in the Child Development Center several years ago, the services of a child and adolescent psychiatrist were found to be of great value in working with some families and their children who had developmental problems.

RECOMMENDATIONS

The World Health Organization (1946) Preamble to the Constitution of the WHO Constitution notes that using triangulated qualitative and quantitative data collection and analysis procedures is viewed as a strength for evaluation research focused on adolescents. This author would add and recommend that these techniques be used for children of all age groups, and particularly for children who are technology dependent and receiving care at home. WHO (1946) also notes that intervention activities that facilitate and promote parent-child relationships and discussion are essential. This author recommends that educators, researchers, and practitioners design interventions that determine the best approaches to implement this activity and the quality of life for children who are technology dependent and their families.

There are multiple definitions of quality of life. Basically, when one considers quality of life, physical, social, and psychological aspects of one's life and existence are considered. The WHO definition of health (1946) is a state of complete physical, mental quality of life, and social well-being and not merely an absence of diseases. It is recommended that cultural diversity dimensions also be considered.

In methodological consideration of measuring quality of life, Faulkner (1999) notes the importance of maintaining a life-span approach, since neurodevelopmental impairments transcend childhood into adulthood. It is not easy to measure quality of life. Quality of life may be experienced differently by different people because of their cultural-subjective experience.

Components of appropriate care for children who are technology dependent and cared for in their homes are case management, respite care, and developmental/educational services. Finances to assure that these services are provided are essential if they are to be a reality. The report to Congress by the Task Force on Technology Dependent Children (1988) statement of consensus agreed that case management with a specified case manager is a component of appropriate care. The report defines service coordination as a process that

- promotes the effective and efficient organization and utilization of medical, social, educational, and other resources to achieve or maintain the maximum potential of the child in the most appropriate and least restrictive environment;
- is community-based and family centered and provides a single service coordinator for each patient and family;
- emphasizes comprehensiveness of services and continuity of care;
- involves active advocacy on behalf of the child;
- is characterized by excellent communication among providers, payors, the child, family, and community;
- ensures a multidisciplinary team planning process that includes the family and is reviewed regularly and on an "as needed" basis; and
- includes quality care assurances and appropriate monitoring evaluation mechanisms.

Whether professional caregivers or a family member assumes the role of case manager, the above aspects of coordination are recommended.

Respite care also was seen as a priority component of appropriate care. It was seen as a service to the family in their caregiving role that provides temporary relief on a planned or unanticipated basis. Respite care is an important resource in home care of a child who is technology dependent and is recommended.

A developmental/educational service is the third component of appropriate care the Task Force identified. Appropriate developmental/education services should be provided to the child in whatever setting the child is at any given time. Services should be planned specifically to each child's capability and potential and are recommended as a vital resource.

There are multiple other factors that must be considered in the care of children who are technology dependent in their homes. The care depends heavily on social and environmental factors in addition to the medical factors. Thus, it is recommended that holism be promoted in the caring for these children and their families. The American Holistic Nurses Association (AHNA) (2000) has developed standards of holistic nursing practice. The standards reflect five core values: holistic philosophy; ethics, theories, and research; nurse self-care; communication, therapeutic environment, and cultural diversity; and holistic caring process. The potential efficacy of these standards may be useful to nurses as they provide support and care to family caregivers and children who are technology dependent. The American Academy of Nursing Task Force on Children has drafted Health Care Quality and Outcome Indicators (2002). In one of the values, it is indicated that holistic health care is integrated into assessment, communication, diagnosis, outcome determination planning, and use of interventions. One of the assumptions specifically notes that health that is holistic includes social, physical, mental, and spiritual dimensions of the child's family. These consumer-oriented indicators should be useful to nurses as they provide health care services to all children and their families.

The President's Advisory Commission on Consumer Protection and Quality in Health Care Industry (1998) identifies four types of quality-related problems: avoidable errors, underuse of services, overuse of services, and variation in practice.

IMPROVEMENT OF QUALITY

As the health care industry becomes more consumer driven it seems all aspects of it will continue to improve. Those agencies providing services to technology-dependent children and their families in the home may find that services will likely improve if the following basic principles are applied:

- Help children and their families host realistic expectations.
- Provide children and families with adequate and appropriate information.
- Demonstrate courtesy, respect, and caring attitudes toward the child and families.
- Be responsive to needs of the children and families.
- Determine if the child and family are satisfied with the care they receive.

The commitment to quality of health care organizations that serve children who are technology dependent and their families starts with the individuals they serve. The next step is to commit to doing everything they want to do better. Bennett and Tibbitts (1989) list a number of traps that should be avoided in the quest for quality improvement. A few of those traps on their list are

- emphasizing scale economies rather than customer concerns
- looking for instant solutions
- placing emphasis on capturing the consumer rather than producing a better product
- concentrating on cost-cutting efficiencies that can be quantified rather than adding to product or service value
- failing to listen carefully and flexibly to provide the service customers genuinely want (and need)
- failing to define quality from the consumers point of view
- failing to support a massive education process needed to cause a major change in attitudes
- having little or no idea of quality's true dimensions
- failing to involve workers and not communicating well-defined, highly visible goals to the individual employee

SUMMARY

Quality care of children who are technology dependent and cared for at home is reflected to some extent in the processes that are in place before the family takes the child home and in the delivering and monitoring of the care once the child is home. The importance of and limitations of outcomes, the use of professional performance standards, the use of evidence-based practice, and the complexity of the families and the variables associated with the different categories of children who are technology dependent are all factors that should be considered and understood when dealing with quality care. Nurses have as a challenge the continued improvement of quality through practice, education, and research.

REFERENCES

Abdellah, F. G., & Levine, E. (1994). *Preparing nursing research for the 21st century.* New York: Springer.

Agency for Health Care Policy and Research (AHCPR). (1998). *Outcome, utilization, and access measures for quality improvement* (AHCPR Publication No. 09-0036). Washington, DC: Department of Health and Human Services.

American Academy of Nursing Task Force on Children. (2002). *Health Care Quality and Outcome Indicators.*

American Holistic Nurses Association. (2000). *AHNA Standards of Holistic Practice: Guidelines for caring and healing.* Gaithersburg, MD: Aspen.

Baldwin-Meyers, A. A., & Oppenheimer, E. A. (1996). Quality of life and quality of care data from a 7 year pilot project for home ventilator patients. *Journal of Ambulatory Care Management, 19*(1), 46–59.

Bennett, A., & Tibbitts, S. J. (1989). *Maximizing quality performance in health care facilities.* Rockville, MD: Aspen.

Collier, A. (2000). Legislation targets errors, safety; center would develop standards. *Worcester Telegram & Gazette.*

Doheny, M. D., Cook, C. B., & Stappen, M. C. (1997). *The discipline of nursing. An introduction* (45th ed.). Stamford, CT: Appleton & Lange.

Faulkner, M. S. (1999). Quality of life for persons with developmental disabilities including commentary by Podilla, S. V. *Scholarly Inquiry for Nursing Practice, 13*(3), 239–256.

Institute of Medicine. (2000). *To err is human: Building a safer health care system.* L. T. Kohn, J. M. Corrigan, & M. S. Donaldson (Eds.). Washington, DC: National Academy Press Committee on Quality Care in America.

Institute of Medicine. (2001). Crossing the Quality Chasm: A new Health System for the 21st Century. Washington, DC: National Academy Press.

Neale, J. E. (2001). Patient outcomes: A matter of perspective. *Nursing Outlook, 49,* 93–99.

Neuman, B. (1995). *The Neuman Systems Model* (3rd ed.). Stanford, CT: Appleton & Lange.

Orem, D. (1991). *Nursing concepts of practice* (4th ed.). St. Louis, MO: C. V. Mosby.

Parker, M. E. (Ed.). (1993). *Patterns of nursing theories in practice.* New York: National League for Nursing Press.

President's Advisory Commission on Consumer Protection and Quality in Health Care Industry. (1998). *Quality first: Better health care for all Americans. Final Report to the President of the United States.* Washington, DC: President's Advisory Commission on Consumer Protection and Quality in the Health Care Industry.

Riehl, J. P., & Roy, C. (1974). *Conceptual models for nursing practice.* New York: Appleton Century Crofts.

Rogers, M. E. (1990). Nursing science unitary, irreducible human beings: Updated 1990. In E. A. M. Barrett (Ed.), *Visions of Roger's Science Based Nursing.* New York: National League for Nursing Press.

Steiber, S. R., & Krowinski, W. J. (1990). *Measuring and managing patient satisfaction.* Chicago: American Hospital Publishing.

Smith, C. E. (1996). Quality of life and caregiving in technological home care. In J. J. Fitzpatrick & J. Norbeck (Eds.), *Annual Review of Nursing Research, 14,* 95–118.

Task Force on Technology Dependent Children. (1988). Report to Congress. Washington, DC.

Wakefield, M., Maddox, P. J., & Bull, J. (2000). 2000 ANA House Delegates Background. Washington, DC: American Nurses Association.

Wamboldt, M., & Wamboldt, F. (2000). Role of the family in the onset and outcome of childhood disorders: Selected research findings. *Journal of American Academy of Child Adolescent Psychiatry, 39*(10), 1212–1219.

Watson, J. (1979). *Nursing: The philosophy and science of caring.* Boston: Little, Brown.

Watson, J. (1988). *Nursing: Human sciences and human care.* New York: National League for Nursing Press.

Wenzel, R. P. (Ed.). (1992). *Assessing quality health care perspectives for clinicians: Historical perspectives.* Baltimore: Williams & Wilkins.

Williams, R., & Yanoshik, K. (2001). Can you do a community assessment without talking to the community? *Journal of Community Health, 26*(4), 233.

Worcester Telegram & Gazette

World Health Organization. (1946). Preamble to the Constitution of the World Health Organization Constitution. Geneva, Switzerland: World Health Organization.

Part III

Strategies for Health Care Providers

Chapter 9

Assessing Growth, Development, and Function

T he child and the family's ecological and cultural (ecocultural) world are defined by the immediate setting—the home and the major institutions or agencies as they directly or indirectly affect them. Families are very important to the developing child whether the child is sick or well. Families matter in every aspect of children's lives. Palfrey (1997) notes that the more we understand about children's health, the more we recognize the delicate intertwining of child and family development. Sameroff and Friese (1990) indicate that children develop through the unfolding of their genetic characteristics in transactions with the environment. They use coping to manage these transactions. Children evolve from a state of dependence as infants to more interdependence and autonomy. The interactions the child has with his/her environment helps the progression of developing cognitive, motor, affective, and communication skills.

The home environment seems to be critical in the development of children (Bradley & Caldwell, 1982; Elardo & Bradley, 1981). Bradley and Caldwell (1976) delineate the relationship between early environment and cognitive development, suggesting that parents play a significant role in organizing the environment for their children. The Early Childhood Home Scale has been used to assess the home environment of various groups of children. Caldwell (1999) developed a supplement to the Early Childhood Home Scale for children living in impoverished urban environments. Health care practitioners, researchers, and educators will likely find that the scale has value in judging the suitability of the home environment before young children who are technology dependent are discharged home, as well as after the child has been placed in home for care.

The effect of chronicity on the developing child is expressed in terms of deficits or developmental lag in the areas of psychosocial, academic, and physical attributes (Holaday, 1984; Wasserman, 1984). The impact of technology dependence on development is difficult to generalize. Findings of Leonberg et al. (1998) from a study on children on prolonged parenteral nutrition (PN) suggest that children who require prolonged PN in early life are at risk for abnormalities in growth, and nutritional status in later childhood; they require long-term dietary, growth, and nutritional monitoring. The degree to which the child's potential development is affected may vary from individual to individual. Patterns may be evident based on profiles that will provide insight into how technology dependence influences development from a perspective of adaptive behavior.

Children ages 7 to 10 years with type 1 diabetes were studied to determine if insulin pump therapy at nighttime, only when children are at home, could improve fasting and nighttime glucose levels without adverse effects. Kaufman, Halvorson, Kim, and Pitukcheewanont (2000) conclude that nighttime-only insulin pump therapy may be a viable alternative that young children can use when they are not under direct supervision of their parents to improve glycemia. Majnemer, Riley, Birnbaum, Greenstone, and Coates (2000) conducted a study to determine if children with severe bronchopulmonary dysplasia (BPD) who required home oxygen therapy were at a greater risk for neurological and motor deficits at school age than preterm peers without BPD. Their findings underline the importance of preventing the cardiorespiratory complications associated with chronic lung disease to minimize disability in preterm children. Better recognition and subsequent remediation of neuromotor impairments that manifest at school age may help maximize their functional potential.

Members of the family and the quality of their lives are expected to be influenced by the child who is technology dependent. Reactions of siblings vary. Some may resent, feel guilty, or overcompensate for the technology-dependent child. The age of the siblings and their understanding of the condition may be important in determining the effect on them. Parental means of discipline and communication patterns influence reactions of siblings (Fleming & Sabatino, 1973). Based on experiences of the author, healthy siblings of children with disabilities or long-term illnesses have a profound effect on the well sibling's life. The illness experience may result in positive or negative consequences for the healthy siblings. Positive effects are reflected in comments that indicate an increased caring, sensitivity, and empathy for the ill child. This tends to enhance the siblings' maturation and promotes greater family cohesion.

While there is evidence of case and anecdotal material, there appears to be a limited number of studies that specifically study the fathers or siblings in terms of the family experience in caring for a technology dependent child in the home. This is an area where more definitive knowledge is needed to assure that quality care is provided to all family members.

In normal development, children from birth to age 19 move through three stages of development: infancy and early childhood, middle years, and adolescence. There are distinct behaviors and skills that are evident in the child in each of these stages of development (Havighurst, 1953). Recognition of these various stages of development provides a guideline for the development of technology-dependent children.

Developmental specialists like Erickson, Lewin, and Piaget have provided insight regarding principles of development (Thomas & French, 1985). Senn and Solnit (1968) have delineated behaviors that suggest problems in development not only of the child or youth but also of the parent. A key to understanding the development of an individual child is the nature of the child's relationship to parents and other primary caregivers. The Barnard Model is based on the assumption that caregivers and children have certain responsibilities to keep the interaction going. Critical to the success of any interaction is the ability of the caregiver and child to adapt to each other (Barnard, Booth, Mitchell, & Telzrow, 1988; Barnard, Hammond, Booth, Mitchell, & Spieker, 1989; Barnard & Kelly, 1990). Barrera and Vella (1987) considered the interactions of disabled and nondisabled infants with their mothers.

Children who have long-term health problems may express themselves differently than other children (Fleming, 1974, 1986; Fleming & Sabatino, 1973). Their developmental needs are likely to differ from those of unaffected children and the developmental needs of the family. Identifying this fact and helping professionals become aware of this may aid work with parents and facilitate the development of strategies that will enhance the quality of life for the child and his/her family.

CONCEPTS IMPORTANT TO DEVELOPMENT

Caring, a difficult concept to translate into measurable terms, was defined by Blattner (1981) as the interactive process by which the nurse and client help each other grow, actualize, and transform toward higher levels of well-being. Watson (1979) identifies several elements of care. Among them are acceptance of the expression of positive and negative feelings, nonverbal warmth, genuineness, and empathy. Some of the elements seem important to facilitating the development of children and youths who are technology dependent and being cared for in the home. Caring seems to be an important concept in the facilitation of development in children and their families.

Social support, stress, coping, and other factors are likely to affect the response of the family caregiver in terms of handling the developmental needs of the child. Studies done on mechanisms of social support of families with special-needs children reflect that social support for families is important (Sabbeth & Leventhal, 1984). The presence of adequate support may be highly predictive of improved family coping. Crnic, Greenberg, Ragozin, Robinson, and Basham (1983) examined the relationships of stress and social support to maternal attitudes. Geary (1989) found that perceived social support of mothers caring for babies on apnea monitors increased over time, but the support network consisted of few individuals, mostly relatives. In another study of mothers of children with chronic versus life-threatening illnesses, larger social networks and more perceived support were reported by the mothers whose children had chronic life-threatening conditions.

HOME CARE AND DEVELOPMENT OF CHILDREN

For home care of pediatric patients to be successful, the developmental, psychosocial, and special health needs of the children as well as the family's needs for support and role modeling must be addressed.

Family development is important in the child's development. Duvall (1971) describes two major phases of the family life cycle that provide a basis for understanding family development. She refers to the first one as the expanding family, which takes the family from its inception to the time the children are grown and leave home. She refers to the second as the contracting family stage, in which children are being launched by the family into lives of their own. The six basic developmental tasks of the family that Duvall (1977) describes and that were presented earlier in this book are essential dimensions to the growth, development, and functioning of children receiving care in their home.

Stein and Jessop (1984) conducted home interviews with 219 families enrolled in a pediatric ambulatory treatment program to evaluate the home care program. Individuals were interviewed three times—at enrollment, six months, and one year. Findings indicate that home care is effective in improving the satisfaction with care and the child's psychological adjustment, and in lessening the psychiatric symptoms of the mother. The conclusion drawn is that home care can be an effective intervention in minimizing social and psychological consequences of chronic illness.

FUNCTIONAL HEALTH STATUS

Functional health status measures in nursing for research, clinical practice, and policy development are important dimensions of development because of the changing health care system. Nurses often are responsible for assisting patients with maintaining or improving their functional status (Moinpour, McCorkle, & Saunders, 1988). In clinical practice and research, the nurse is often the professional who is involved in obtaining these measures.

To provide a brief overview of functional health status measures in nursing, the following will be addressed:

1. Defining what is meant by functional health status
2. A brief distinction between screening and assessment
3. The need for functional status measures
4. Factors in selecting and administering functional status measures
5. Identifying select measures that are often used or cited
6. Concluding statements.

Practice, research, and policy concerns will be highlighted throughout.

Functional status in nursing may be viewed from the perspective of activities of daily living. Or it may be viewed by physical condition. This would include upper extremity functions, lower extremity functions, sensory functions, excretory functions and mental and emotional status. Functional health may be perceived in terms of communication, nutrition (metabolic), elimination, activity (exercise), sleep (rest), cognition (perception), self-perception (self-concept), role (relationship), sexuality (reproductive), coping (stress tolerance), and values (belief).

The terms "physical functioning," "functional status," and "daily living activities" have been used interchangeably and are sometimes equated with other terms, such as health status, level of impairment, and/or disability. An overlap of what is described as functional capacity activities and daily living activities is apparent. Stein and Jessop (1990) describe Functional Status II as a measure of child health status. Functional Status II is a revision of Functional Status Measure (FSM I), developed in 1978. The authors note that it has particular strengths for the measurement of health status of children with chronic physical conditions who are not disabled.

Carnevali (1988) has defined activities in daily living as encompassing anything that patients, their families, or persons in their immediate network do that is relevant to the presenting health situation. Daily living activities in the broadest sense include eating, sleeping, personal hygiene, and elimination, as well as other activities that affect or are affected by the presenting health situation. Carnevali further notes that functional health status in the nursing domain involves age-related psychobiological status, developmental task status, and functional status as it is affected by pathological and associate medical diagnostic and treatment activities. The policy that physical health assessment be considered an expected aspect of nursing has resulted in the importance of documenting observations made in this regard. Functional health patterns are an example of measures that have become an integral part of nursing documentation.

Because there are varied definitions of functional health status, one of the first issues that should be considered in measuring this phenomenon is a definition of the term. Daily living activities, broadly conceptualized, are inherent in the definitions of functional health status that have been reviewed. Functional health status activities include measurement of an individual's ability to move about physically, maintain body (bathing, dressing, combing hair), ingest food, eliminate waste, and carry out basic social functions of communication and behavior in a manner appropriate to the environment in which the individual exists and the age of the individual.

One thing that seems clear is that functional health status is a major aspect of nursing in primary care. "Health" refers to adaptation to modification of physiological processes to achieve homeostasis. "Equilibrium" refers to maintenance process without significant diminution of physiological or behavioral functioning. Put another way, maintenance of and promotion of appropriate functioning are the basis of primary care. Consequently, instruments that can help health professionals obtain reliable, valid, and sensitive measures of the functional health status of children and members of their families are essential.

Screening vs. Assessment

Screening and/or assessment for functional status, which includes developmental tasks, will enable the nurse to initiate interventions designed to improve functioning. Both concepts are used in research and practice. The essential task in screening is to identify individuals who manifest a high probability of significant deficits. The essential task in assessment is to identify, as specifically as possible, the nature and degree of the difficulty and the domains of residual competence so that assistive intervention may be mobilized to help overcome and/or manage the functional difficulty.

Assessment is one of the aspects of the nursing process in planning and implementing care. Assessing might include using screening measures, as well as more definitive measures. However, it is important to distinguish when a screening instrument is being used as opposed to an assessment instrument.

From a research methodological perspective, patient outcome is a widely accepted measure of health care and, consequently, could be a measure of functional capacity. Another view of nursing outcomes is that they are difficult to find because many cannot be solely attributable to nursing care (Bloch, 1975). These observations are made because nurses usually screen without input from other disciplines. Screening may be viewed as a part of process rather than outcome. However, to carry out an overall assessment of functional health status, it may necessitate involvement of other disciplines in addition to nursing.

Need for Functional Status Measures

Progressive impairments in physical functional abilities contribute significantly to loss of independence and long-term care needs. Basic descriptive data are needed to increase our understanding of impairments and functioning in various cultural groups of families who have children who are technology dependent and to determine needs for appropriate health care and services among these populations. Data are sparse on the relationship of physical frailty to chronic degenerative conditions, particularly in children who are technology dependent from minority populations. Better knowledge of genetic, environmental, nutritional, cultural, and socioeconomic factors affecting the severity and progression of such conditions would be useful in the design of intervention and prevention programs.

Any conditions that affect the functional health status of technology-dependent children in various population groups are important. Cancer, acquired immunodeficiency syndrome (AIDS), arthritis, and some cardiorespiratory conditions are among the diseases that affect the functional health status of a large segment of the population, some of whom may be members of families of children who are technology dependent. Mental health functional status is another concern, particularly among family caregivers of technology-dependent children and the growing homeless and elderly population groups.

Retardation in cognitive abilities, physical growth, and motor abilities and disabilities resulting from other causes are the basis of malfunctioning and maladaptation in some individuals. Delivery of better services to these individuals who are now more visible in our society is being demanded. The challenge is to be able to justify reimbursement based on assessed individual needs. Providers of services are being held accountable to meet the needs in a fiscally responsible manner.

Laws have resulted in policies that require certain functional health status measures. The most prominent example of this was the Supreme Court's decision in *Zebly v. Sullivan*. The 1990 Supreme Court decision emphasized the need for individualized assessment of a child who applies for Social Security Act Supplemental Security Income Benefits if that child has an impairment or a combination of impairments comparable in severity to one that would disable an adult. The court ruled that although a vocational analysis is inapplicable to children, this does not mean that functional analysis cannot be applied to them through an inquiry into the impact of an impairment on the normal, age-appropriate daily activities of the child, such as speaking, walking, washing, dressing, feeding, going to school, playing, and all the other activities in which children normally engage. Nurses, as well as other health professionals, could be involved in the individualized assessments needed to make the determination as to whether the child who applies for benefits receives them or not.

The Omnibus Budget Reconciliation Act of 1986 ordered the development of the Uniform Needs Assessment Instrument for Post-Hospital Discharge. The instrument is used to evaluate the needs of patients for post-hospital extended care services, home health services, and long-term care services of a health-related or supportive nature. Evaluation of individual functional capacities and the nursing and other care requirement necessary to meet health care needs to assist the patient in living with functional incapacities would be done.

With more assessments being done in the home for the technology dependent or assisted and other home-bound ill persons, nurses likely will play an even greater role in measuring functional health status. Multiple policy issues need to be considered in addressing the need for functional status measures: How often should one be assessed, and by whom? Should one receive benefits based on functional status measures? Should functional status measures be used to place individuals in levels of care in nursing homes and other community services?

Some of the major causes of interferences in "normative" functioning involve two critical questions: (1) Should a person's first contact in any given episode of illness or potential illness with the health care system lead to a decision of what must be done to help resolve the person's problem? and (2) Is there responsibility for the continuum of care (i.e., maintenance of health, promotion of health, and prevention of health problems)? These dimensions are important to consider in primary care. Measures are needed to determine functional health status initially, as well as over time. The issue of labeling and its benefits and deficits may be resolved with using measures over time.

FACTORS IN SELECTING AND ADMINISTERING TOOLS

A key factor in selecting a measurement tool of functioning is to determine its effectiveness in assessing ability and capacity and its overall appropriateness for use with the patients who are to be assessed. Prior information about the patient or group of patients and the present status of the patient or group of patients are important factors that the nurse or person administering the tool must consider.

Sensitivity of the instrument to measure phenomena in the particular group of patients is often overlooked in selecting an appropriate tool. Caution to assure the instrument is a sensitive one, as well as reliable and valid for the group of patients being studied or evaluated clinically, cannot be overstated. Investigators should consider which groups were used to establish the instrument's reliability and validity.

Questions need to be raised as to how sensitive a tool is to minority populations—Hispanic, black, and Asian—considering the growth expected in minorities in the next decade. Sociological research suggests that class, not race, may be a key factor in disease rates. Increasingly, some health experts are questioning the orientation to race and urging the consideration of class in measuring health status. Zigler and Hall (2000) express concern about the health care of American children. They note that there is a powerful (if indirect) link between poverty and disorders in mental health.

Differences found may be the result of race, biological differences, and lifestyle factors. These may contribute to health problems, along with disadvantages such as poor diet and reduced access to care that afflict the poor, regardless of their color.

In assessing functional health status, data that would provide a standard for evaluating the current status of the individual are important. Individuals could be compared with others of their own sex, or their status could be measured by their own functioning. In other words, they become their own control.

Variation in examiners affect the creation of a desirable test environment. The examiner needs to be aware of the nuances that may affect results in administering, scoring, and interpreting the instrument. The length of the scale, acceptability, and cost also are important considerations in selecting an instrument for use in research and practice. If a tool is too long, it will not be practical to try to use it. Other factors that are not direct measures of proper physiological functioning, such as stress, environment, family functioning, and involvement in planning and implementing therapeutic regimens, are critical and may affect the patient's response. They are among those factors with which nurses are usually knowledgeable.

Figure 9.1 is a list of assessment instruments that may be used with technology-dependent children. (See Appendix at end of chapter for information on where instruments can be obtained.) The Stein and Reissman (1980) Impact on Family Scale instrument, which measures impact on the family of an ill child and has been used by several researchers, is an effective means of obtaining data that will help nurses plan care with parents who are in care giving roles. The Impact on Family Scale has four dimensions from which information about economic consequences for the family (fi-

---

- AAMD Adaptive Behavior Scale
- Bayley Scales of Infant Development
- Beck Depression Scale
- Bender Visual Motor Gestalt Test
- Bright Futures Guidelines
- Cain-Levine Social Competency Scale
- CES-D Scale
- Child Behavior Checklist (CBCL)
- Denver Developmental Screening Test (DDST)
- Developmental Assessment for Severely Handicapped (DASH)
- Family APGAR Scale
- Feetham Family Functioning Survey
- Functional Status II
- Home Observation for Measurement of the Environment
- Impact on Family Scale
- Neonatal Behavior Assessment Scale
- Nursing Child Assessment Feeding Scale
- Nursing Child Assessment Teaching Scale
- Vineland Adaptive Behavior Scale (VABS)

FIGURE 9.1   Instruments that can be used in studying and/or caring for children who are technology dependent and their families.

For more information about these instruments, see Appendix at end of chapter.

nancial burden) disruption of social interaction, personal strain (psychological burden) experienced by the primary caretaker, and the coping strategies (mastery) employed by the family can be identified. The scale has been used effectively in studies of chronic childhood illnesses. The across-culture study by Kolk, Schipper, Hanewald, Casari, and Fantino (2000) is the most recent report noted where the scale was used.

Caldwell's (1999) Home Scale, which measures the home environment, has been updated. This instrument is used often by nurses. The assessment of the home environment includes a general assessment and specific areas related to the client's age and health status. The general assessment involves the nurse's observation of potential hazards, safety, and basic comfort needs (such as whether the home is heated/cooled at a comfortable level, availability of hot water, sanitation, the cleanliness of the environment, whether the home is a warm loving environment, etc.). The specific age-related areas are assessed in terms of influence on the child's development, safety, parent-child interaction, appropriate health care, discipline, and so forth. For example, the Home Observation for Measurement of the Environment (the birth to 3 years version) has six categories: (1) emotional and verbal responsivity of parent; (2) avoidance of restriction and punishment; (3) organization of physical and temporal environment; (4) provision of appropriate play material; (5) parental involvement with child; and (6) opportunities for variety in daily stimulation. Each category has a number of items for which a "yes" or "no" response can be made following the observation.

Feetham (1991) delineated concepts on measures of family dynamics and methodological issues in research of families. The Family Function Survey provides perceptions of family members and is another tool that can be used by nurses (Feetham & Humenick, 1982). Nurses may find these individual instruments and ideas useful in considering a holistic approach to working with families.

Small and Schutz (1990) ask the question, what are the biological and environmental factors that contribute to gender and differences in physical performance? Thomas and French (1985) acknowledge that biology plays a salient role in increasingly large gender differences. They propose that environmental factors assume even greater importance following puberty.

Carrying out a functional assessment of an individual family depends on the functional areas that are to be assessed. Gordon (1987) identifies functional health patterns as

- Health perceptions—health management related to general health management and prevention practices

- Nutritional—metabolic, elimination
- Activity—exercise
- Sleep—rest
- Cognitive perception—self concept
- Role relationship
- Sexuality—reproductive
- Coping—stress tolerance and value belief

There are various instruments, techniques, and approaches that will help health professionals assess physiological functions, the patterns described by Gordon, growth and development, family functioning, etc. The professional that carries out functional assessments must consider the norm for the attribute being assessed. The professional must be skilled in carrying out physiological assessments and obtaining psychosocial information from individuals being assessed. The professional should use interviewing where appropriate as a means for getting information and must be a skilled interviewer. Observation and listening skills are essential if one is to be an effective assessor of functioning. Following the instructions carefully in administering the various tools or using information provided from other professionals who have administered tests or scales requires care as the information from functional assessments often will be used in planning care for the child.

The major means of obtaining data about functional status is through clinical assessment, self-report, use of inventories and specific instruments, and actual observation. Obtaining a complete database on health status functioning is important. Rehabilitation and habilitation are two processes that may emerge as potential outcomes from developing plans based on the assessment of functional health status.

Measures of functional health status, to some extent, are dependent upon the age-appropriateness of the measure. This is particularly true for children. Measures for children may be more difficult to obtain than for older individuals. Experimental control is more difficult to maintain because behavioral change over extended intervals of time is the phenomenon that is being studied in developmental research of children. The nurse can assess the child from a clinical nursing perspective and/or use standard inventories of behavioral or physical ramifications that interfere with normal functioning. Measurement of change and the rate of change may be a critical observation. If retrospective data are used, the problems of selective forgetting and purposeful and/or unconscious distortion of the data may result. Developmental studies that provide indicators of functional status are likely to include repeated and frequent measures.

Time is another factor that should be considered. A report of a 1986 audit of 150 randomly selected radiation therapy patient records revealed that 147 records contained a complete nursing assessment and weekly progress notes. Concern was expressed about the amount of time spent in documenting without jeopardizing detailed information obtained in the initial nursing assessment (Deyer, Macher, & Radovich, 1990). A pilot test was done of a patient self-assessment tool based on Gordon's (1987) functional health pattern nursing assessment and the use of a flow sheet that contained both frequently used nursing diagnoses and potential intervention. The findings showed that both subjective and objective information had improved. Documentation of time was reduced and the information more comprehensive (Hirshfield-Bartek, Dow, & Creton, 1990).

Sampling considerations also are important in carrying out developmental studies because of the concern with trying to ensure that normative statements about children in terms of their age are explained. It is also necessary to explain the nature of differences between the age groups.

Motivation, desire, and expectation based on health beliefs certainly may be a factor in individuals' functioning. Bandura (1977b) defined self-efficacy as an individual's conviction that her or she is capable of executing the behaviors necessary to provide a desired outcome. Successful mastery experiences result from bolstering efficacy expectations. Efficacy cognitions and causal attribution in a social or therapeutic feedback context suggest potential intervention, as well as other experimental studies.

Other Select Measures

In addition to tests and scales mentioned earlier in the chapter, a few other measures are noted here and in Figure 5.1 from which information can be obtained that would be useful to nurses in working with families and their children. To screen and/or assess general development in children there are several often cited instruments used by nurses.

Bayley Scales of Infant Development (BSID)

These scales cover the age range of 2 months to 30 months. BSID comprises a mental scale and motor scale designed to measure sensory-perceptual behavior and coordination of large muscles and fine motor control, respectively. In addition to the two scales, there are 30 behavior ratings. The authors report that on the mental scale, the items having both high test-retest and high tester-observer reliability were those dealing with object-oriented behavior. Highly reliable items in the motor scale are those concerned with independent control of the head, trunk, and lower extremities.

Denver Developmental Screening Test (DDST)

This is a popular screening test designed to screen four developmental areas: personal-social, fine motor-adaptive, language, and gross motor in children ages 0 to 6 years. The mean examiner observer reliability for items included in the Denver II is .99 with a range of .95–1.00. The test-retest reliability of the same items is .90 with a range of .50–1.00. For the DDST, test-retest ranged from .90% to 1.00%. Reliability among examiners on the percent of agreement on items passed or failed ranged from 80% to 95%.

Neonatal Behavior Assessment Scale

This is a popular motor assessment instrument that nurses find useful in testing organized behavioral and neurological responses of newborns to environmental events and the use of state behavior. The instrument has 47 scores—27 behavioral items and 20 elicited items. Data are not normed. Several reliability studies have been done. An unwieldy amount of information is collected. There is some evidence for predictive validity. The test-retest reliability using agreement by two criterion was .796 for males and .850 for females.

Vineland Adaptive Behavior Scale

This is a revision of the Vineland Social Maturity Scale, which assesses presocial and social functioning. Information is obtained through semi-structured interviews. There are 13 scores. Split-half and test-retest reliability coefficients for the survey form range from .83 for the motor skills domain to .94 for the composite. Interrater coefficients range from .62 to .78.

Nursing Child Assessment Teaching Scale (NCATS)

The Nursing Child Assessment Teaching Scale is a reliable and valid means of observing and rating caregiver-child interaction for the purpose of assessing whether a dyad has problems in interaction and communication patterns. The teaching scale is organized into six subscales representing 73 items. Four subscales describe the caregiver's behavior and responsibility to the interaction: sensitivity to cues, response to distress, social-emotional growth fostering, and cognitive growth fostering. Two subscales describe the child's behavior and responsibility to the interaction: clarity of cues and responsiveness to the caregiver. The scale is appropriate for children from birth to 36 months. The teaching scale is scored following the observation of a session in which the caregiver is asked to teach the child a standardized age-appropriate task. Length of teaching varies, but generally ranges from 1 to 6 minutes. Materials needed to conduct the observation include a teaching manual, teaching kit, and scale. NCATS is widely used in research and clinical practice with families and young children. To use the teaching scale, professionals must be trained through the NCATS programs and be certified (reliable) in the use of the scale.

Nursing Child Assessment Feeding Scale

The Nursing Child Assessment Feeding Scale contains a well-developed set of observable behaviors that describe caregiver-child communication and interaction during the feeding situation from birth to 12 months. The scale is organized into six subscales representing 76 items. Four subscales describe the caregiver's responsibility to the interaction: sensitivity to cues, response to distress, social-emotional growth fostering, and cognitive growth fostering. Two subscales describe the child's responsibility to the interaction: clarity of cues and responsiveness to caregiver.

The scale is scored following an observation of a feeding episode, which can include breast, bottle, or solid feedings. The length of feeding varies with the age of the child and the type of feeding. Materials needed to conduct the observation include a feeding manual and scale. The scale has been used in several studies. It demonstrates high internal consistency of the total score, parent score, infant score and the parent contingency score. The test-retest reliability is better for the parent items than infant. To use the feeding scale, professionals must be trained through the NCATS programs and be certified (reliable) in the use of the scale.

There are a number of other measurements being used by health professional in practice and research, including nurses, to assess and screen children's developmental functioning. Among them are the APGAR Score, the Developmental assessment for Severely Handicapped, the Bender-Visual Motor Gestalt Test, the Cain-Levine social Competency Scale, Stein, Reiseman and Jessop's Functional Status II and the AAMD Adaptive Behavior

Scale to name a few. Many of the scales used to measure developmental functioning in children are incremental, in that the oldest children being measured in a study would have the broadest or most comprehensive responses. The Bright Futures Guidelines for Health Supervision of Infants, Children and Adolescents provide some achievement tasks for the family and health supervision outcomes for the specific developmental period. They can be used for developmental surveillance and milestones, for parent/child interactions and anticipatory guidance.

The following are highlights from the Bright Futures Guidelines (Green, 1994):

- Health supervision consists of those measures that help promote health, prevent mortality and morbidity, and enhance subsequent development and maturation.
- Health supervision goals include enhancing families' strengths, addressing families problems promoting resiliency, building parental competence, and helping families share in the responsibility for preventing illness or disability and promoting health.
- Health supervision requires a partnership between health professionals and families.
- Health supervision is shaped primarily by issues raised by the parent and child, with their expectations, questions, and concerns addressed.
- Health supervision involves assessing the strengths and issues for a specific child, family, and community. Health supervision includes the interview, the physical examination, observation of the child and family, and psychosocial, educational, and developmental surveillance.
- Health supervision that employs specific preventive and health-promoting interventions leads to improved outcomes. The social developmental and health outcomes occur along a continuum, varying in their timing from child to child and family to family.
- Because health risks and needs can change over a period of weeks or months, they need to be reassessed periodically.
- The benefits of continuing health supervision are best ensured by a medical home offering health services that are accessible, continuous, comprehensive, family-centered, coordinated, compassionate, and integrated into a system of care.
- Health supervision can be provided in many settings, often with collaboration between a variety of organizations and disciplines.
- Health supervision helps educate children and families about the efficient use of health care and other community services.

- Child development serves as the basic science for much of health supervision, especially health promotion.
- Special populations such as those with chronic illness or disability will require more health supervision.
- Supplemental health supervision may also be needed during periods of family transition or stress.

SUMMARY

Anyone planning to use the tools described in this chapter to obtain measures of development or health status functioning should evaluate the latest available psychometric data on each of the tools. If more than one rater is involved, it is important to establish interrater reliability. It would be wise to consider factors that affect results. There are ethical as well as policy issues that are important to consider. Development and functional health status measures constitute a set of information that allows for making multiple decisions about children and their families, such as where and by whom they will be cared for and who will be paid to document the status and provide this information to make decisions about the patient. Permission of the health care provider to collect the data and disseminate it becomes an issue in informed consent.

Resources are finite but information or knowledge is not. Therefore, how best to obtain and use the knowledge about developmental and functional health status measures in the context of resources available is another policy issue that needs to be addressed.

The importance of further defining what is meant by developmental and functional health status cannot be overemphasized. Finally, there are other factors that are not necessarily directly related to development and function health status but that may affect responses of individual children. How to enhance the quality of life of children who are technology dependent and assure humane consideration of them may be determined by developmental and functional health status measures. Health policy decisions should not be based solely on how one performs on such measures, but on a combination of factors that affect the individual.

APPENDIX

Resources for Obtaining Assessment Instruments

AAMD Adaptive Behavior Scale
Authors: Kazvonihira, Ray Foster, Max Shellhaas, and Henry Leland

This scale is designed to measure children's personal independence and social skills. Adaptive behavior is defined as the effectiveness or degree to which the individual meets the standards of personal independence and social responsibility expected for his or her age and cultural group. It is used/recommended as part of classification/diagnostic battery in screening and placement decisions regarding the mentally handicapped, ages 3 to adults.

Publisher: Publishers Test Service
             Order Services Center
             P.O. Box 150
             Monterey, CA 93942–0150
             Phone: 800–538–9547
             Fax: 800–2282–0266

Bayley Scales of Infant Development (BSID)
Author: Nancy Bayley

The test is designed to assess the developmental functioning of infants 1 to 42 months of age. Three subscales make up the test: mental scale, motor scale, and behavior rating scale.

Publisher: The Psychological Corporation
             555 Academic Court
             San Antonio, TX 78204–2498
             Phone: 800–211–8378
             Fax: 800–232–1223

Beck Depression Inventory
Author: Aaron T. Beck

This 21-item inventory measures the level of depression in adults. It assesses the severity on an individual's complaints, symptoms, and concerns related to the current level of depression. A number of symptoms are assessed. Questions are presented at an eighth-grade level.

Publisher: Center for Cognitive Therapy
             133 South 36th Street, Room 602
             Philadelphia, PA 19104
             Phone: 215–898–4200

Bender Visual Motor Gestalt Test (BVMGT)
Author: Lauretta Bender

The test is designed to measure perceptual motor skills. It intends to determine visual-motor gestalt functioning in children, neurological maturation, and organic brain defects. The test can be administered to an individual child ages four years up or in a group.

Publisher:　The American Orthopsychiatric Association, Inc.
　　　　　　19 West 44th Street
　　　　　　Suite 1616
　　　　　　New York, NY 10036
　　　　　　Phone: 212–564–5930
　　　　　　Fax: 212–564–6180

Bright Futures: Guidelines for Health Supervision

The Bright Futures Guidelines for children and adolescents, birth through 21 years of age, cover four developmental sections and provide specific information on health supervision tailored specifically to infancy, early childhood, middle childhood, and adolescence. The guidelines were updated and revised in 2000.

National Center for Education in Maternal and Child Health, Georgetown University.

Cain-Levine Social Competency Scale
Authors: Leo F. Cain, Samuel L. Levine, and Freeman F. Elzey

The scale measures social competency of trainable mentally retarded children. It consists of 44 items of four aspects of social competence: self-help, initiative, social skills, and communication. Percentile norms based on children who are mentally retarded are offered for chronologically ages 5 through 13 years.

Publisher:　Consulting Psychologist Press
　　　　　　577 College Avenue
　　　　　　P.O. Box 60070
　　　　　　Palo Alto, CA 94306

Center for Epidemiologic Studies–Depression (CES-D) Scale

This scale measures symptoms associated with depression in adults. Questions deal with symptoms of depressed mod, lack of energy, insomnia and appetite loss.

Publisher:　Epidemiology and Psychopathology Research Branch
　　　　　　Division of Clinical Research

National Institute of Mental Health
5600 Fishers Lane, Room 10C–05
Rockville, MD 20857
Phone: 301–443–4513

Child Behavior Checklist (CBCL)
Authors: Thomas H. Achenbach and Craig Edelbrock

The test is designed to assess the behavioral problems and social competencies of children through the use of ratings and reports by different informants. The child's behavioral problems are evaluated from four perspectives. Children ages 4 to 18 can be assessed.

Publisher: University Associates in Psychiatry
1 South Prospect Street
Burlington, VT 05401
Phone: 802–656–4563
Fax: 802–656–8747

Denver Developmental Screening Test (DDST)
Author: William K. Frankenburg

This test is used to detect developmental delays during infancy and the preschool years. Four main categories are assessed: personal–social development, fine motor adaptive development, language development, and gross motor development.

Publisher: LADOCA Project and Publishing Foundation, Inc.
East 51 Avenue and Lincoln Street
Denver, CO 80216

Developmental Assessment for the Severely Handicapped (DASH)
Author: Mary Kay Dykes

The purpose of this test is to provide a discrete profile of the child's functioning levels of skills across socioemotional, language, sensorimotor, activities of daily living, and preacademic areas. The test is designed for individuals functioning within the developmental range of birth to 8 years.

Publisher: Pro-Ed, Inc.
8700 Shoal Creek Blvd.
Austin, TX 78758–6897
Phone:800–897–3202
Fax: 800–397–7633

Family APGAR
Author: G. Smilkstein

This screening tool consists of questions designed to reflect a family member's satisfaction with the functional state of the family.

Journal of Family Practice, 6(6), 1231–1978.

Feetham Family Functioning Survey
Authors: Suzanne Feetham and S. Humrenick

This survey provides information about family members' perception of relationships that contribute to or are affected by family function.

Functional Status II (FSII)
Authors: Ruth E. K. Stein and Dorothy Jones Jessop

This measure is designed to assess the health status of children 0 to 16 years. The FSII has both a long (43-item) and a short (14-item) version. The long version consists of general health and stage specific factors for each age group. The short version uses a common core of items across the entire age span.

Medical Care, November 1990, Vol. 28, No. 11, pp. 104–1055.

Home Observation for Measurement of the Environment
Authors: Betty Caldwell and Robert Bradley

The purpose of this inventory is to assess the quality and quantity of support for cognitive, social, and emotional development available to a child in the home environment. There are three versions of this inventory: infant and toddler, early childhood, and middle childhood.

Publisher: Center for Research on Teaching and Learning
College of Education
University of Arkansas at Little Rock
33rd and University
Little Rock, AR 72204
Phone: 501-569-3422

Impact on Family Scale
Authors: Ruth E. K. Stein and K. Reissman

The scale is a 24-item questionnaire that measures four dimensions of impact: financial burden, familial/social impact, personal strains, and mastery.

Dr. Ruth Stein
Department of Pediatrics
Albert Einstein College of Medicine of Yeshiva University
Montefiore Medical Center
111 East 210th Street
Rosental Pavilion
Bronx, New York
Phone: 718–920–6490

Neonatal Behavioral Assessment Scale
Author: T. Berry Brazelton

This scale is used to examine newborn behavior. It is being used by clinicians to sensitize parents to the capacity of their newborn. A new edition of the manual provides pertinent information on the scale and administration of each item and criteria for scoring.

Publisher: Cambridge University Press
             Edinburg Building
             Shaftesbury Road
             Cambridge, England CB2 2RV
             Phone: 44(0)22223312393
             Fax: 44(0)1223315052

Nursing Child Assessment Feeding Scale
Nursing Child Assessment Teaching Scale
Author: Kathryn Barnard

These scales are developed around six constructs of caregiver-child interaction. Four constructs pertain to caregiver: sensitivity to cues, response to distress, socioemotional growth, and cognitive growth fostering. Two subscales pertaining to the child are clarity of cues and responsiveness to the caregiver. The Feeding Scale covers ages birth to 12 months of life, and the teaching scale is appropriate for children from birth to 36 months.

Publisher: NCATS Programs
             University of Washington
             P.O. Box 357920
             Seattle, Washington 98195–9720
             Phone: 206–543–8528

Vineland Adaptive Behavior Scale (VABS)
Authors: Sara S. Sparrow, David A. Balla, and Domenie V. Cicchett

The purpose of this test is to provide a general assessment of adaptive behavior. It assesses the social competence of individuals. It requires that a respondent familiar with the behavior of the individual in question answer behavior orientation questions posed by a trained examiner of children and youth ages birth to 18 years.

Publisher: American Guidance Service
4201 Woodland Road
Circle Pines, MN 55014–1796
Phone: 800–328–2560
Fax: 612–786–9077

REFERENCES

Apgar, V. (1966). The newborn Apgar scoring system: Reflections and advice. *Pediatric Clinics of North America, 113*, 645–650.

Bandura, A. (1977a). *Social learning theory.* Englewood Cliffs, NJ: Prentice-Hall.

Bandura, A. (1977b). Self-efficacy: Toward a unifying theory of behavior change. *Psychological Review, 8*, 191–215.

Barnard, K. E., Booth, C. L., Mitchell, S. K., & Telzrow, R. W. (1988). Newborn nursing models: A test of early intervention to high-risk infants and families. In E. S. Hibbs (Ed.), *The psychological aspects of the family.* Toronto: Lexington Books.

Barnard, K. E., Hammond, M. A., Booth, C. L., Mitchell, S. K., & Spieker, S. J. (1989). Measurement and meaning of parent-child interaction. In F. J. Morrison, C. E. Lord, & D. P. Keating (Eds.), *Applied development psychology, Vol. III.* New York: Academic Press.

Barnard, K. E., & Kelly, J. F. (1995). Assessment of parent-child interaction. In S. J. Meisels & P. Shonkoff (Eds.), *Handbook of early childhood intervention* (pp. 278–302). New York: Cambridge University Press.

Barrera, M. E., & Vella, D. M. (1987). Disabled and non-disabled infants' interactions with their mothers. *American Journal of Occupational Therapy, 41*, 168–172.

Beya, S., & Matzo, M. (1989). Assessing elders using the Functional Health Pattern Assessment Model. *Nurse Educator, 14*, 32–37.

Blattner, B. (1981). *Holistic nursing.* Englewood Cliffs, NJ: Prentice-Hall.

Bloch, D. (1975). Criteria, standards, norms—crucial terms in quality assurance. *Journal of Nursing Administration, 7*(7), 20–30.

Bradley, R., & Caldwell, B. (1976). Early home environment and changes in mental test performance in children ages 6 to 36 months. *Developmental Psychology, 12*, 93–97.

Bradley, R., & Caldwell, B. (1982). The consistency of the home environment and its relation to child development. *International Journal of Behavioral Development, 5*, 445–465.

Caldwell, B. (1999). Development of a supplement to the Home Scale for Children Living in Impoverished Urban Environments. *Journal of Developmental and Behavioral Pediatrics, 18*(5), 329–330.

Caldwell, B. M., & Boyd, J. W., Jr. (1984). Effective marketing of quality child care. *Journal of Children in Contemporary Society, 17*(2), 25–36.

Carnevali, D. (1988). Daily living and functional health status: A perspective for nursing diagnosis and treatment. *Archives of Psychiatric Nursing, 2,* 330–333.

Cassel, J. (1974). Psychosocial processes and stress: Theoretical formulations. *International Journal of Health Services, 4,* 471–482.

Crnic, K. A., Frederich, W. N., & Greenberg, M. T. (1953). Adaptation of families with mentally retarded children. A model of stress, coping, and family ecology. *American Journal of Mental Deficiency, 88,* 125–138.

Crnic, K. A., Greenberg, M. T., Robinson, N. M., & Ragozin, A. S. (1984). Maternal stress and social support: Effects on the mother-infant relationship from birth to eighteen months. *American Journal of Orthopsychiatry, 54*(2), 224–235.

Deyer, B., Macher, N., & Radovich, H. (1990). Functional health patterns in the post anesthesia care units approach to identification. *Journal of Post Anesthesia Nursing, 5,* 157–162.

Duvall, E. M. (1971). *Family development.* Philadelphia: J. B. Lippincott.

Duvall, E. M. (1977). *Marriage and family development.* Philadelphia: J. B. Lippincott.

Edwardson, S. R. (1988). Revision and testing of the Hussmann and Hegevary outcome measure for myocardial infarction. Measurement of nursing outcome. In C. Waltz & O. L. Strickland (Eds.), *Measuring Client Outcomes* (pp. 24–37). New York: Springer.

Elardo, R., & Bradley, R. (1981). The home observation for measurement of the environment: A review of research. *Developmental Review, 1,* 113–145.

Erickson, E. H. (1963). *Childhood and society.* New York: W. W. Norton.

Feetham, S. L. (1991). Conceptual and methodological issues in research of families. In A. L. Whall & J. Fawcett (Eds.), *Family theory development in nursing. Sociological science and art.* Philadelphia: F. A. Davis.

Feetham, S. L., & Humenick, S. S. (1982). The Feetham Family Functioning Survey. In S. S. Humenick (Ed.), *Analysis of current assessment strategies in the health care of young children and childbearing families* (pp. 259–267). Norwalk, CT: Appleton Century Crofts.

Fitzmaurice, K., & McLean, H. A. (1997). A computer-generated test of acuity for multihandicapped children. *Australia and New Zealand Journal of Ophthalmological Supplies, 1*(5), 9–11.

Fleming, J. (1974). Hospitalized physically disabled children focus on things, not people. *Perceptual and Motor Skills, 39,* 1002.

Fleming, J. (1981). An evaluation of the use of the Denver Developmental Screen Test. *Nursing Research, 30,* 290–293.

Fleming, J., Holmes, S., & Stephens, L. (1988). Differences in color preferences of school age children in varying stages of health. *Maternal Child Nursing Journal, 17*(3), 173–189.

Fleming, J., & Sabatino, D. (1973). Children's drawings aid researcher in understanding health and conditions. *Nursing Research Reports, 7,* 5–6.

Geary, P. A. (1989). Stress and social support in the experience of monitoring apneic infants. *Clinical Nurse Specialist, 3,* 119–125.

Gladwell, M. (1990, November 26). Public health experts turn to economic ills. *The Washington Post,* p. A3, Science final edition.

Green, M. (Ed.). (1994). *Bright Futures Guidelines for Health Supervision of Infants, Children and Adolescents.* Arlington, VA: National Center for Education in Maternal and Child Health.

Havighurst, R. S. (1953). *Human development and education.* New York: Longmans, Green.

Healey, A., Keesee, P., & Smith, B. S. (1989). *Early services for children with special needs: Transactions for family support.* Baltimore: P. H. Brookes.

Hirshfield-Bartek, J., Dow, K. H., & Creton, E. (1990). Decreasing documentation time using a patient self-assessment tool. *Oncology Nursing Forum, 17,* 251–255.

Holaday, B. (1984). Challenges of rearing a chronically ill child: Caring and coping. *Nursing Clinics of North America, 19*(2), 361–368.

Kahn, L. (1984). Ventilator-dependent children heading home. *Hospitals, 58,* 54–55.

Kaufman, F. R., Halvorson, M., Kim, C., & Pitukcheewanont, P. (2000). Use of insulin pump therapy at nighttime only for children 7–10 years of age with type I diabetes. *Diabetes Care, 23*(5), 579–582.

Kolk, A. M., Schipper, J. L., Hanewald, G. J. F. R., Casari, E. F., & Fantino, A. G. (2000). The Impact on Family Scale: A test of invariance across culture. *Journal of Pediatric Psychology, 25*(5), 323–329.

Leonberg, B. L., Chuang, E., Eicher, P., Tershakovec, A. M., Leonard, L., & Stallings, V. A. (1998). Long-term growth and development in children after home parenertal nutrition. *Journal of Pediatrics, 132,* 461–466.

MacElveen-Hoehn, P., & Eyres, S. (1984). Social support and vulnerability: State of the art in relation to families and children. In B. Raff, K. Barnard, & P. Brandt (Eds.), *Families of vulnerable infants* (Vol. 20, pp. 11–43). New York: March of Dimes Birth Defects Foundation.

Majnemer, R., Riley, P., Birnbaum, R., Greenstone, H., & Coates, A. L. (2000). Severe bronchopulmonary dysplasia increases risk for latent neurological and motor sequelae in preterm survivors. *Developmental Medicine and Child Neurology, 42*(1), 53–60.

Maskowitz, E. (1957). *Pulse profile.* Elmsford, NY: Pergamon Press.

McGarth, J. (1970). *Social and psychological factors in stress.* New York: Holt, Rinehart and Winston.

Moinpour, C. M., McCorkle, R., & Saunders, J. (1988). Measuring functional status. In M. Frank-Stromburg (Ed.), *Instruments for clinical nursing research* (pp. 23–45). Norwalk, CT: Appleton and Lange.

O'Pray, M. (1980). Developmental screening tools: Using them effectively. *Maternal Child Nursing, 5,* 126–130.

Palfrey, J. S. (1997). Family matters. *Bright Notes, 2*(3). Washington, DC: U.S. Department of Health and Human Services Administration, Public Health Service.

Sameroff, A. J., & Friese, B. H. (1990). Transactional regulation and early intervention. In S. J. Meisels & P. P. Shonkoff (Eds.), *Handbook of early childhood intervention* (pp. 119–149). Cambridge, MA: Cambridge University Press.

Sabbeth, B., & Leventhal, J. (1984). Marital adjustment to chronic childhood illness: A critique of literature. *Pediatrics, 73,* 762–767.

Scott, D., Oberst, M., & Dropkin, M. (1980). A stress coping model. *Advances in Nursing Science, 3,* 9–23.

Senn, M., & Solnit, A. (1968). *Problems in child behavior and development.* Philadelphia: Lea Lebiger.

Small, F. L., & Schutz, R. W. (1990). Quantifying gender differences in physical performance: A developmental perspective. *Developmental Psychology, 26,* 360–369.

Stein, R., & Jessop, D. J. (1984). Does pediatric home care make a difference for children with chronic illness? *Pediatrics, 73,* 545–552.

Stein, R., & Jessop, D. J. (1990). Functional Status II: A measure of child health status. *Medical Care, 28,* 11, 1041–1055.

Stein, R., & Reissman, C. (1980). The development of an Impact on Family Scale: Preliminary findings. *Medical Care, 18,* 465–471.

Thomas, J. R., & French, R. E. (1985). Gender differences across age in motor performance: A meta-analysis. *Psychological Bulletin, 98,* 260–282.

Thomas, R. M. (1985). *Comparing theories of child development.* Belmont, CA: Wadsworth.

Wasserman, A. (1984). A perspective study of the impact of home monitoring and the family. *Pediatrics, 74,* 325–329.

Watson, J. (1979). *Nursing: The philosophy and science of caring.* Boston: Little, Brown.

Zigler, E., & Hall, N. W. (2000). *Child development and social policy theory and application.* New York: McGraw-Hill.

Chapter 10

Case Management

C ase management programs offer comprehensive services, new care options, and coordination of care to technology-dependent children with complex needs (Deeming & Wolf, 1997; Miller, Rice, Deibe, & Fos, 1998). Case management is a problem-solving strategy for helping people arrive at key decisions about their lives (Grisham, White, & Miller, 1983). It has also been described as a collaborative model of community nursing practice that seems to be an effective means of providing care to children who are technology dependent and cared for in the home by their families (Campbell, 1998; Chan & Fillippone, 1998). According to Barkauskas (1990), it is vital that nurses who care for patients in their homes, who assume leadership in home care, and are the largest group of professionals in the field, provide high-quality care. Callahan (1981) notes that the goal of case management is helping people within the limits of available resources.

Case management services have been defined as services to promote the effective and efficient organization and utilization of resources to ensure access to necessary comprehensive services for patients, in this case children and their families. Case management appears to be an important dimension in providing home care to children who are technology dependent. Inherent in the concept of case management is the notion that children who are technology dependent and their families need help with the coordination of problems that may arise that are medical, psychosocial, developmental, educational and/or environmental (American Academy of Pediatrics, 1984). The case manager, who often is a nurse, is responsible for coordinating the services of other providers, such as the physical and occupational therapist, social worker, and educators involved in providing care to the child and the family. Mullahy (1998) presents the role of the case manager as varied. Some of the roles they assume are coordinators, facilitators, impartial advocates, and educators. Their titles and specific duties depend on where they are employed.

Case management and managed care are confusing; some people think they are interchangeable concepts, but they are not. Case management is a personalized process that aims to identify high-risk or high-cost patients, assess treatment options and opportunities to coordinate care, design treatment programs to improve quality and efficiency of care, control costs, and manage patient care to ensure the optimum outcome (Mullahy, 1998). Managed care basically is a system of cost-containment programs. Case management may be a component of managed care strategy.

The case manager must be an effective communicator and attend to legal and ethical responsibilities. The chapter on Legal and Ethical Responsibilities of the Case Management Profession in Mullahy (1998) is very informative, and readers of this book are encouraged to read it.

Lamb (1995) provides an excellent critique of the cumulative body of knowledge on case management intervention inside and outside of nursing. She notes that the literature on nursing case management is rich with description. Two of the common themes across nursing case management practice, according to Lamb, are that nurses functioning as case managers work with individuals, families, and populations at high risk to adverse health outcomes, and those nurses are responsible for applying the nursing process in ways that potentially enhance both quality and cost outcomes. While there is a deficit of theory-based research in the case management of children who are technology dependent and cared for in their home, there is enough knowledge about case management generally that warrants consideration of intervention strategies (Chamberlin & Rapp, 1991; Ethridge & Lamb, 1989; Lamb, 1992; Lamb, 1995; Redford, 1992). Insights and knowledge of nurses based on their experience in working with technology-dependent children need to be reported in the literature, as other nurses may be able to use the strategies and approaches in providing care to these children and their families (Radford, Thorne, & Bassingthwaighte, 1997).

Storgion and Stutts (2000) note that advances in medical knowledge and technology have created two populations of technology-dependent children: those who wean off support while they are hospitalized and those who require long-term support. The latter group basically is seen as those who receive care in their home. Health professionals provide these children with technical care, psychosocial development support, education for their families, and coordination of multidisciplinary care. Storgion and Stutts see case management as the means to meet the challenge of providing care through individualized and multidisciplinary plans to children with available reimbursement funds.

DISCHARGE PLANNING

Boosfeld and O'Toole (2000) note that for successful discharge planning, collaboration between all professionals involved is essential. They discuss seven specific steps:

1. Needs assessment (not only immediate needs but also long-term needs of the family rather than on a short-term crisis intervention)
2. Identification of key workers
3. Discharge proposal (a comprehensive report detailing information regarding the child's medical and social history, his or her needs for future care, a plan for discharge and follow-up care, and a list detailing all equipment and ongoing costs involved)
4. Multidisciplinary planning meetings
5. Recruitment and selection of a home care team
6. Training
7. Moving home

Before a child who is technology dependent is discharged from the hospital to home care, it is essential and logical that the child is medically stable. Patient factors, family factors, community factors, and the child's disease process and medical stability are determinants in the feasibility of discharge to home care (American Academy of Pediatrics, 1984).

The interdisciplinary team will depend on what the child's needs are. Parental involvement in the discharge plan is essential to its success.

Both external and internal factors influence the quality and effectiveness of home care and are critical to the success of home care. The internal factors include parental abilities and attitudes. External factors include the availability of professional nurses prepared in high technology home care or pediatric home care, and, where indicated, the availability of other health care professionals and the quality of the equipment available. There are likely to be quality of care issues in the home that do not or rarely arise in the hospital. Astute professionals will be prepared to address these issues.

Discharge planning is a critical factor in preparing families before the child goes home. Specific dimensions of discharge planning in addition to those noted by Boosfeld and O'Toole (2000) that should be considered are (1) a determination as to what agency will be selected for home care if there are choices, (2) who from that agency will be assigned to the family, and (3) who will serve as the case manager. It is important that the family knows what can and cannot be expected from the home health care agency.

Case management is viewed as essential because it is usually the case manager's role to help the family set realistic goals, participate in the care planning, measure outcomes, help the family with coping strategies, solve problems related to the delivery of care, help with communication with other members of the multidisciplinary team, and function in accordance to the Case Management Society of America (CMSA) standards of practice for case management (CMSA, 1995). The CMSA delineates standards of care required for safe and effective case management and standards of performance, including quality of care, legal/ethical advocacy issues, resource utilization, and research.

The care task of case management is to determine the client's most suitable residence and to marshal the services that will enable the client to return to or to remain in the residence (Grisham, White, & Miller, 1983). The complexities involved in home care are (1) the condition of the child is fluid as the child's needs change, and (2) the partnership between the parents and health care professionals is an integral part of the child's life, considering that the family is an integral part of the child's life.

Key issues in case management, according to Grisham, White, and Miller (1983), are staffing, case load, supervision, leadership, targeting, accountability, management, liability, and subjectivity in decision making. The importance of documentation of care to provide uniform information cannot be overstated.

Prior to discharge, transitional care may be necessary. Storgion and Stutts (2000) note that the literature on case management, children dependent on technology, and family issues provides the conceptual framework for the development of a case management base unit. They describe a study done to assess the efficacy of a transitional unit. A retrospective chart review was done to collect data from 10 ventilated patients who made up the convenience sample. The results indicated that there was a decrease in daily costs and hospital stay and that a cohort of patients for rehabilitation therapies as well as training registered nurses, patient care assistants, parents, and volunteers in the delivery of the services decreased the need for additional therapists. Length of stay also decreased significantly. Effective communication and collaboration among all care providers was seen as important in meeting the patient's discharge needs with the least amount of misinformation, confusion, and hospital readmissions. Once the child is discharged and is receiving care in the home, nurses may use whatever conceptual schema they feel most comfortable with in implementing the nursing process and determining the home care of technology-dependent children.

McCoy and Votroubeck (1990) provide a system approach to pediatric home care. Chapters are devoted to alterations in neurological, respiratory, cardiac, metabolic, endocrine, and renal functions. Their approach covers developmental issues and family considerations. King, King, and Rosenbaum (1999) note that family-centered care involves ensuring that parents have ultimate control over decision-making, treating parents of children with disabilities respectfully and supportively, and providing them with needed information. They studied linking the caregiving process with outcome. Their findings suggest that better caregiving leads to parents being more satisfied with services, which in turn leads to less stress. Such findings support the importance of case management in helping with the delivery of family-centered caregiving.

Case management helps to facilitate family-centered care. The nurse often is the coordinator of care from the other health care professionals who interact with the family. Consequently, the nurse-family relationship must be a positive one if the delivery of home care to the child who is technology dependent is going to be effective. The nurse-parent collaboration is based on definitive communication strategies between the nurse and the parent. Berlin and Fowkes (1983) describe the LEARN Model for use by nurses in collaborative problem solving. They identify LEARN as

L = Listen with . . . understanding to the family's perception of the problem

E = Explain your perception of the problem

A = Acknowledge and discuss differences and similarities

R = Recommend treatment

N = Negotiate agreement

The National Center for Family-Centered Care of the Association for the Care of Children delineated nine elements of family-centered care. Among them were recognition that the family is the constant in a child's life; honoring racial, ethnic, cultural, and socioeconomic diversity of families; recognizing family strengths and individuality; and respecting different methods of coping. The professionals who keep these elements in mind are likely to be very effective in assessing and working with families in implementing care of their children.

To effectively manage the care of children who are technology dependent and cared for in the home, several of the classifications of client's problems addressed by community nurses that follow may be helpful. The classification and a client management system for community health nursing agencies published by the U.S. Department of Health and Human Services is available through National Technical Information Service, 5285 Port Royal Road, Springfield, VA 22161—NTIS Accession #HRP0907023. A modified version to illustrate how nurses may use the domains follow.

CASE MANAGEMENT ASSESSMENT TOOLS

Domain 1. Environment

Income

> Deficit—Is the inadequacy of income to cover expenses incurred because of medical or health-related needs of the technology-dependent child?
> Supporting statements—"Mother quit her job last month as she did not have anyone to stay with child who has to have intravenous feedings." Signs and symptom?

Lowered Income

> Potential deficit—The child may need intravenous feedings at home longer than the health insurance will cover.
> Health promotion—The mother wants guidance in budgeting and managing money and information.

Sanitation

> Deficit—Sanitation is designated as a problem when a sign/symptom of inadequate storage for intravenous feedings is noted. Sign/symptom: discoloration of feeding.
> Potential deficit—May be the review labels on feedings and contact company that supplied them.

Residence

> Deficit—Focuses on living quarters of child who is technology dependent and on oxygen several hours a day. Sign/symptom: inadequate space to accommodate oxygen apparatus.

Potential deficit—Nurses who care for children who are technology dependent and their families must carry out the following functions:

1. Assessment: This requires that the nurse obtain information through appropriate means, including interview, observation, physical examination, review of records, etc.
2. Diagnosis: Identify the problem(s) after analyzing the information.
3. Develop a plan of care: Goals are set to handle the problem(s) identified. The goals may be prioritized and stated as short- and long-term goals.
4. Carry out the plan: The implementation of the strategies may need to be modified as the nurse executes the plan.
5. Evaluation: Continuous evaluation is a part of the process. The need to document actions is a legal responsibility, and the written plan including evaluation should be available to the family and to third-party payers if needed. The information should reflect updates and changes made to provide care.

Domain 2. Psychosocial

Communication with Community Resources

Impairment—Identifies the signs/symptoms that reflect the caregiver's difficulty or frustration when using complex community service systems. Sign/symptom: unfamiliar with options/procedures for obtaining services, may be appropriate for statements such as "does not know how to apply for social security supplement," or "cannot find sitter to stay with child when needed."

Social Contact

Impairment—Relates to the caregiver. Database information such as "new to community and has not made friends" may suggest the sign/symptom of limited social contact.

Potential impairment—Caregiver diagnosed as depressed.

Health promotion—Caregiver concerned about relationships with parents of children who are disabled.

Role Change

Impairment—Evolves from situations in which the independent member of a unit becomes dependent, or vice versa. It is also appropriate for clients who assume an additional role before completing the developmental tasks of the current role. Assumes additional role(s) could relate to parents of a child who requires an apnea monitor at home.

Potential impairment—Parents expected a healthy first-born child but have a child that requires monitoring.

Health promotion—Parents are concerned about the effects the child's condition will have on all of their lives.

Interpersonal Relationship

Impairment—Suggests difficulty in a significant relationship. For example, the relationship may involve a husband and wife. Sign/symptom: minimal shared activities evidenced by "husband's job that necessitates that he travel" or wife complains about his never being home and that she has the responsibility for all child care.

Potential impairment—History of three divorces.

Health promotion—Couple expresses interest in learning common pitfalls in husband/wife relationships when there is a child who is technology dependent.

Spiritual Distress

Actual—Is associated with stress caused by challenges to beliefs, values, culture, or religion. The database may suggest the sign/symptom, disrupted spiritual rituals, as evidenced by child needs a blood transfusion and the religion does not allow.

Potential impairment—Severe case of anemia from leukemia condition.

Health promotion—Parents are interested in learning what can be done so they can adhere to their religion and yet do what is recommended for their child.

Grief

Impairment—Not limited to grief associated with death. It may be used to describe grief due to other losses, such as amputation of a limb or divorce. The sign/symptom, difficulty coping with grief responses, would be recorded when a child is diagnosed with a renal condition that will require dialysis.

Potential impairment—End-stage renal disease.

Health promotion—Parent interested in learning more about renal dialysis.

Emotional Stability

Impairment—Can be evidenced by a wide range of signs/symptoms. For example, "repeatedly asking the same questions during the visit" may denote the. Sign/symptom: scattering of attention.

Potential impairment—Child recently discharged home and is receiving oxygen.

Health promotion—Caregiver expresses interest in learning relaxation techniques.

Human Sexuality

Impairment—Focuses on attitudes and feelings related to male-female roles. Normal psychosexual maturation includes a healthy self-concept and integration of the overt and covert aspects of sexuality into the individual's life. Sign/symptom: difficulty expressing intimacy since child has been home with a nose gastric tube; wife complains of sexual needs being ignored by spouse.

Potential impairment—Mate.

Health promotion—Parents ask how to inform.

Caretaking/Parenting

Impairment—Reflected in situations occurring in the family caring for a child who is technology dependent. The parent or the child may exhibit the sign/symptom, dissatisfaction/difficulty with responsibilities, by the statement, "I can't take another day with this situation."

Potential impairment—Grandparents come to live with family, including young children.

Health promotion—Young woman requests a home nursing course.

Growth and Development

Impairment—Is not appropriate for a 4-year-old child. The sign/symptom, age-inappropriate behavior, applies to "4-year-old boy continues to wet the bed regularly."

Potential impairment—An 8-month-old child who is technology dependent is at 80th percentile for weight.

Health promotion—Knowledgeable parents of a 2-year-old child who is technology dependent request information on growth and development.

Domain 3. Physiological

Hearing

Impairment—Abnormal results of hearing screening test are noted through standardized or formal methods, such as a whisper test or observations of the community health nurse and family members.

Potential impairment—Child has frequent ear infections.

Health promotion—Parent interested in anatomy and physiology of ear in relation to infant care.

Vision

Impairment—Child squints and holds objects close. This information suggests the. Sign/symptom: difficulty seeing objects.

Potential impairment—Child has strabismus.

Health promotion—Caregiver interest in lighting conducive to seeing items better.

Speech and Language

Impairment—Focuses on the skills that facilitate verbal communication. The child seems to have a receptive speech impairment and demonstrates the sign/symptom of abnormal ability to understand or respond appropriately.

Potential impairment—Child's mother is deaf.

Health promotion—Parents request information regarding teaching the child to speak.

Dentition

Impairment—Sign/symptom: teeth growing crooked of a child on home ventilation.

Health promotion—Nurse asks to discuss with family the need for the child to see a dentist.

Cognition

Impairment—May be used for an 8-year-old child who seems to be developing slowly mentally. The nurse's recording, "seems to not be aware of the days of the week" may suggest the sign/symptom disorientation to time.

Potential impairment—Normal development of mental abilities.

Health promotion—Mother and nurse develop exercises for the child, which will enhance orientation to time/place person.

Consciousness

Impairment—Is a problem label and modifier particularly useful with a terminally ill client. "Rarely shows any response" or "does not acknowledge voices of family members" suggest the sign/symptom of unresponsiveness.

Potential impairment—Diagnosis of cancer.

Health promotion—Caretaker requests information regarding coma.

Integument

Impairment—May be used with many types of skin problems. The sign/symptom, rash, could be reflected by "diaper area reddened" or "cries when diaper is wet."

Potential impairment—Infection of edematous skin.

Health promotion—Young teenage girl being cared for in home expresses concerns about skin care and use of makeup.

Neuromusculoskeletal Function

Impairment—Includes the sign/symptom of decreased muscle strength, which may be noted when the database states "unable to walk without assistance."

Health promotion—Young adult on home care wants to go to clinic for physical therapy.

Respiration

Impairment—Is described by a cluster of signs/symptoms, which include coughing. A database may state, "reports coughing episode almost every morning."

Potential impairment—Caregiver has smoked two packs of cigarettes daily for 10 years.

Health promotion—Client expresses interest in stopping smoking.

Circulation

Impairment—May be used with the caregiver who "complains of swollen legs." She may demonstrate the sign/symptom, edema, when she describes a history of swollen legs.

Potential impairment—Family history of hypertension.

Health promotion—Young adult caregiver seeks information for low-cholesterol diet.

Digestion-Hydration

Impairment—Results from disease or disturbances, which affect the gastrointestinal tract. Sign/symptom: child's stools with blood and mucus.

Potential impairment—Child taking additional vitamins and minerals for chronic ulcerative colitis.

Health promotion—Caregiver concerned about relation between stress and ulcer and ulcerative colitis.

Bowel Function

Impairment—The sign/symptom of abnormal frequency/consistency of stool may be evidenced by the infant who is having "four liquid stools daily."

Potential impairment—History of occasional constipation.

Health promotion—Caregiver requests information regarding high-fiber diet.

Genito-Urinary Function

Impairment—The sign/symptom, incontinent of urine, is suggested by "bed wet at time of dressing change" or "Foley catheter continues to leak."

Potential impairment—History of bladder infections.

Domain 4. Health-Related Behaviors

Nutrition

Impairment—Child on parenteral nutrition.

Potential impairment—Not able to maintain use of parenteral nutrition because of cost.

Health promotion—Caregiver compares caloric and nutritional value of IV nutrition.

Sleep and Rest Patterns

Impairment—Includes the sign/symptom of insufficient sleep/rest for age/physical condition. The database of a young caregiver may state, "is tired from demands of caring for child who is technology dependent."

Potential impairment—Up to check on child two or three times at night.

Health promotion—Caregiver asks about relationship of rest to health.

Physical Activity

Impairment—May be used for clients of all ages. The sign/symptom, inappropriate type/amount of exercise for age/physical condition, suggests exercise that is either excessive or deficient for the client's status.

Potential impairment—Works full-time as a word processor.

Health promotion—Caregiver wants help with developing an exercise program for child and self.

Personal Hygiene

Impairment—Reflects a lack of generally accepted standards of cleanliness. Dirty clothing may be noted on the record with, "wearing the same clothes as last week."

Potential impairment—Diagnosis of neglect.

Health promotion—School nurse asked to talk to child and caregiver about using soap, shampoo, and deodorant.

Prescribed Medication Regimen

Impairment—Includes "deviates from prescribed dosage," when the caregiver "admits forgetting to give child medications occasionally."

Potential impairment—Caregiver may be exhibiting signs of undue stress.

Health promotion—Parents ask about recommended immunizations for child.

Technical Procedure

Impairment—Involves the caregiver's ability to perform a procedure or treatment, such as an injection or urinary catheter irrigation. The client may not be able to perform the procedure or treatment after instructions are provided by the community health nurses, thus the sign/symptom, unable to demonstrate/relate procedure accurately, is appropriate.

Potential impairment—Introduction of infection.

Health promotion—Caregiver asks for information about techniques used for irrigating catheter.

SUMMARY

The concept of case management and its practice appears to be a valued approach to caring for patients/clients in diverse practice settings. It is a means of providing care for patients/clients across the continuum of care. Its use in the care of children who are technology dependent and being cared for in their homes is an important aspect of care. The process of case management continues to be dynamic and viable for practicing nurses and other health care professions. Those involved in case management will recognize the necessity for the multiple considerations that are involved in working with families and caregivers in the delivery of safe, high-quality care of patients and clients. Case manager researchers face critical challenges as health policymakers, administrators, and clinicians look for data to support the use of care management as a central block in the restructured health care system (Lamb, 1995).

REFERENCES

American Academy of Pediatrics. (1984). Task Force on Home Care.

Barkauskas, V. H. (1990). Home care. In J. J. Fitzpatrick, R. L. Taunton, & J. Q. Benoliel (Eds.), *Annual review of nursing research* (Vol. 8, p. 103). New York: Springer.

Berlin, & Fowkes, (1983). A teaching framework for cross-cultural health care. *Western Journal of Medicine, 139*(6), 155–157.

Boosfeld, B., & O'Toole, M. (2000). Technology-dependent children: Transition from hospital to home. *Pediatric Nursing, 12*(6), 20–22.

Callahan, J. (1981). Single agency option for long-term care. In J. Callahan & S. Wallack (Eds.), *Reforming the long-term care system*. Lexington, MA: Lexington Books.

Campbell, T. (1998). Caring for the technology dependent child: A case study. *Nursing Praxis in New Zealand, 13*(2), 5–10.

Case Management Society of America (CMSA). (1995). Standards of Practice for Case Management. Little Rock, AR: CMSA.

Chan, J., & Filippone, A. (1998). High-tech pediatric home care: A collaborative approach. *Caring, 17*(5), 30–36.

Chamberlin, & Rapp, C. A. (1991). A decade of case management: A methodological review of outcome research. *Community Mental Health Journal, 27,* 171–188.

Deeming, L. M., & Wolf, J. C. (1997). Case management for ventilator dependent children. *Journal of Case Management, 3*(5), 15–16, 18, 21.

Ethridge, & Lamb, (1989). Professional nurse case management improves quality, access and costs. *Nurse Management, 20*(3), 26–29.

Grisham, M., White, M., & Miller, L. (1983). Case management as a problem solving strategy. *Journal of Long Term Home Health Care, 2*(4), 21–28.

King, G., King, S., & Rosenbaum, P. (1999). Family-centered caregiving and well-being of parents of children with disabilities: Linking process with outcome. *Society of Pediatric Psychology,* 41–53.

Lamb, G. S. (1992). Conceptual and methodological issues in nurse case management research. *Advances in Nursing Science, 15*(2), 16–24.

Lamb, G. S. (1995). Case management. In J. J. Fitzpatrick & J. S. Stevenson (Eds.), *Annual review of nursing research case management* (Vol. 13). New York: Springer.

McCoy, P., & Votroubeck, W. (Eds.). (1990). *Pediatric home care: A comprehensive approach*. Rockville, MD: Aspen.

Miller, V. L., Rice, J. C., Deibe, M., & Fos, P. J. (1998). The analysis of program and family cost of case management for technology dependent infants with bronchopulmonary dysphasia. *Journal of Pediatric Nursing,*

Mullahy, C. M. (1998). *The case managers' handbook* (2nd ed.). Gaithersburg, MD: Aspen.

Mundinger, M. O. (1984). Community based care: Who will be the case managers? *Nursing Outlook, 32,* 294–295.

National Center for Family-Centered Care of the Association for the Care of Children's Health. Bethesda, MD:

Radford, M. J., Thorne, S., & Bassingthwaighte, C. (1997). Long-term gastrostomy in children: Insights from expert nurses. *Issues in Comprehensive Pediatric Nursing, 20*(1), 35–50.

Redford, (1992). Case management: The wave of the future. *Journal of Case Management*, 1(1), 5–8.

Storgion, S., & Stutts, A. (2000). Transitional care: A multidisciplinary case management-based unit. *Pediatric Nursing*, 26(6), 584–568.

Thorne, S. E., Radford, M. J., & McCormick, J. (1997). The multiple meanings of long-term gastrostomy in children. *Journal of Pediatric Nursing*, 12(2), 89–99.

Chapter 11

Financial Aspects of Care

Home care that combines the latest in medical technology with traditional comfort and security requires services and products limited only by the imagination of medical equipment research and design experts and the willingness of home care personnel to provide the services (Haddad, 1996). Limits do exist, such as the availability of reimbursement for services and products, the capabilities of patients and families, and the very real problem of providing care in an environment that was not originally designed for this purpose. Resources in the form of community and professional services and products in the form of medicine and equipment are vital in providing quality health care to children who are technology dependent and receiving care in their home. The outcome of care is dependent on having finances that make it possible to have these resources available. Information in this chapter may help professionals find innovative means to assist families with the financial aspects of care and/or stimulate ideas for future research.

FINANCIAL CONSIDERATIONS IN HOME CARE

Financial resources to purchase and maintain equipment, to construct home facilities if needed, and to obtain the professional help that is necessary to care for the child in the home are things that must be carefully planned before the child is discharged home. Boosfeld and O'Toole (2000) note that particularly for ventilator-dependent children, the package can be very expensive. They also note that questions about suitable medical treatment are generally decided by looking at relative costs, including risks and benefits. An economic evaluation of health care using a cost-benefit, cost-effectiveness, or cost-utility analysis, they note, is often criticized for being subjective and biased or for not including morals and values.

Costs for care in the home are for the most part viewed as lower than costs for care in the hospital. What most of the cost studies do not show is the unseen costs to families that result. It is necessary to evaluate direct and indirect costs for any child who is technology dependent and cared for in the home during the discharge planning stage and periodically thereafter. As the child grows and develops, the care status is likely to change as family members also are changing.

Cost is a constant issue for almost every parent who has a chronically ill child. Few data are available to reflect costs specifically for chronically ill children. Hobbs, Perrin, and Ireys (1985) categorize costs by initial identification and evaluation, initial treatment, continuing treatment, special service needs, and daily care routine. Such factors as increased electricity bills and costs of equipment maintenance are not listed by Hobbs, Perrin, and Ireys, but they are essential considerations in the overall cost of home care.

Pless (1974), in discussing theoretical and practical considerations in the measurement of outcomes, notes that "an outcome is achieved only by the expenditure of some limited resource. The resources on the input side include money (which may be the most important), manpower, time, and the energy and attention of the family. The relationship between a given input and an outcome is unlikely to be linear. There is no reason to believe that by spending $1,000 rather than $100 on a particular therapy, the outcome will be 10 times better. It is even possible that there maybe no direct relationship between a particular input and an intended outcome" (Pless, 1974, p. 6).

Varricchio (1994), in addressing home care for cancer patients, raises several important issues and poses relevant research questions. Although she does not specifically discuss the child who is technology dependent, she notes that human and indirect costs must be considered in establishing overall costs. Indirect costs and human costs are paid out of pocket or are related to psychological morbidity; they also are related to psychological and health-related burdens of the caregiver and to loss of income to caregivers (who in the case of children usually are parents).

The various sources of payment relate in a complicated fashion, making the true family economics of chronic disability complex. Quantifying the contribution that the family provides to care in the home would add tremendously to the knowledge base of care in the home. Glendinning, Kirk, Guiffrida, and Lawton (2000) assessed available data on the numbers of technology-dependent children living at home in the United Kingdom and the estimated costs of caring for them. They found that all existing sources of data had some shortcomings and concluded that routine information on the numbers of technology-dependent children discharged home was urgently needed so that consideration could be given to the high cost of services.

When the family takes the child home, the caregiving costs associated with home care technology include direct financial expenditures and indirect costs in the loss of employment and psychosocial drain (Smith, 1995). Direct costs are substantially more than institutional care. Costs were saved by third-party payors, not by family caregivers. Holdsworth et al. (1997) concluded from an examination of the economic impact of a home chemotherapy program for pediatric oncology patients that the program resulted in substantial monetary savings to third-party payers.

Parette (1993) found that the cost of sustaining children can be high, depending on the extent of the child's need and type of equipment required. According to Smith (1996), a number of researchers have found that costs of caregiving in the home to those who depend on technology relate to a number of factors, including hours per day of care, years of caring, and the relationship between the caregiver and the patient. The various sources of payment relate in a complicated fashion, making the true family economics of chronic disability and dependency on medical technology a complex problem. It is not known whether the cost care package for these children is adequate. Quantifying the contribution of the family in providing care to chronically ill children who are dependent on medical technology would provide valuable information about the cost of care. Further, attempting to unravel some of the complexity relative to the true family economics would be useful in decision-making for care. There are not many examples of innovative approaches. One state, in attempting to use its MCH funds in the most advantageous manner, recommended that the Apnea Monitoring Program be discontinued. This meant that the funds for the rental of apnea monitors would no longer be available but would be available to help mothers with their babies. Priority was given to babies whose mothers were in the prenatal program at 100% or 185% of the poverty level, and babies who were in the Regionalization of Perinatal Care Program (Hernandez, 1986).

Albrecht (1991) considers the reliability and validity of an instrument designed to predict the cost of home care nurse visits based on several factors, including the severity of the client's problems, physical, psychosocial, teaching needs, clinical judgment difficulty, and multiagency involvement based on an analysis of the workload. More longitudinal research and experimental research is sorely needed to ascertain the "real" cost of caring for children who are technology dependent in their home. Using the categories of identifying these children that was established by the

Office of Technology Assessment (1987) may be one means of conducting studies of the costs of home care.

WHO FINANCES HOME CARE
FOR TECHNOLOGY-DEPENDENT CHILDREN?

Medicaid of the Social Security Act is administered by states. It provides financial assistance to dependent children whose families' income or resources are too low to provide necessary assistance. Exactly how each state administers Medicaid for children who are technology dependent to qualifying families varies. Private insurers may also support aspects of home care. It is vitally important that families who want to care for their children who require technology at home to understand what is covered by Medicaid or private insurance. The descriptions of two programs that may provide some financial assistance follow.

Supplemental Security Income (SSI)

The Supplemental Security Income (SSI) program for children, which is administered by the Social Security Administration, is one that can be helpful to parents caring for children who are technology dependent in the home. The program

- provides monthly cash payments based on family income;
- qualifies a child for Medicaid health care services in many states; and
- ensures referral of SSI child beneficiaries into the State Title V Children With Special Health Care Needs Program's system of care.

Under current regulations, the SSA considers a child to be disabled if

- the child has a medically determined impairment (physical or mental) that results in marked and severe functional limitations; and
- the condition has lasted or is expected to last at least a year or is expected to cause death within a year.

Health care providers who encounter families with children who are technology dependent and being cared for at home may wish to tell families about the program and how to apply. The American Academy of Pediatrics

(2001) provides information on how to apply and what to tell families about SSI application, disability determination, and appeals procedures.

To be eligible for SSI, a child must be a U.S. citizen or a naturalized citizen. For SSI disability purposes, a child is an individual who is younger than 18 years of age. Children authorized to remain in the United States by the Immigration and Naturalization Service may also qualify. The child must also reside in one of the 50 states, the District of Columbia, or the Northern Mariana Islands. Children living in Puerto Rico, Guam, and the United States Virgin Islands may be U.S. citizens but do not meet the SSI requirements for residency. The exception is children of military personnel assigned to overseas duty.

How to Apply for SSI Benefits

To apply for SSI benefits for a disabled child, a parent should call the SSA's toll-free number (1–800–772–1213) to make an appointment for a telephone interview or visit an SSA office to complete an application.

If parents make an appointment for a telephone interview, an SSA claims interviewer will contact them. The interviewer will provide general information to parents about the medical, disability, and functional criteria used to determine SSI eligibility. This information is provided to help parents decide whether to proceed with the application process. The SSA prefers that parents use the telephone process because, according to the SSA, it is more efficient for both the parents and the SSA.

Parents need to know the following:

- The telephone line is often busy, but they should keep trying.
- The SSA interviewer will gather information about family income, financial resources, and the child's citizenship.
- On the basis of the gathered information, the interviewer will indicate whether it appears that the child is financially eligible for SSI.
- The interviewer will ask whether the parent or guardian wants to file an application for the child.
- The parent has a right to request and file an application even if it does not appear that the child qualifies financially.
- Application forms completed by phone will be sent by mail to the home for signature.
- The telephone interviewer should not suggest that the child does (or does not) appear to meet the SSI disability criteria.

- The date of the telephone interview serves as the protected filing date, so there is no loss of benefits. A record should be kept of all contacts with the SSA, including the date and phone number with the extension of the person with whom they spoke.
- The process of determining disability can take several months.
- Financial eligibility for young adults 18 years or older is based only on what the young adult owns and/or earns. Family income and assets are not considered.

If parents choose to go to a local SSA field office, they should call either the local office or the toll-free number to make an appointment. This will ensure that an SSA staff person will be available to take the application and will reduce the amount of waiting time when filing an application. If parents cannot gather all of the required information by the time of the appointment, they should still go to the SSA field office at that time to begin the application process, thus establishing a protected filing date. When the SSA has the needed information about family income and financial resources, financial eligibility for SSI will be determined.

State Children's Health Insurance Program (SCHIP)

The need to reduce both financial and nonfinancial barriers so that all children can have health insurance would provide greater access to care for them. The State Children's Health Insurance Program (SCHIP), established as Title XXI of the Social Security Act, provides an expansion of insurance coverage for a large number of uninsured children and is a positive step in ensuring greater access to health care for children. There are three approaches from which states have selected to provide health insurance coverage to children. They are expanding Medicaid, creating or expanding a non-Medicaid children's health insurance program, or a combination of the first two approaches.

SCHIP covers children through 18 years. The American Academy of Pediatrics Committee on Child Health Financing (1998) notes that Congress should expand SCHIP to allow states to include children through 21 years of age. "Reimbursement levels must ensure reasonable clinician compensation in relation to increased time required to coordinate and provide care for children, particularly those with special health care needs" (American Academy of Pediatrics, 1998).

Persons interested in the SCHIP program in their state may get information needed from one of the following numbers. These numbers, most of which are toll-free and are direct ones to the children's health insurance program are listed on the Health Care Financing Web page (www.hcfa. gov.medicaid/obs5.htm).

Alabama: 1–888–373–5437
Alaska: 1–888–318–8890
Arizona: 1–877–764–5437
Arkansas: 1–888–474–8275
California: 1–888–747–1222
Colorado: 1–800–359–1991
Connecticut: 1–800–811–6141
Delaware: 1–800–996–9969
District of Columbia: 1–800–666–2229
Florida: 1–877–316–8748
Georgia: 1–800–934–9206
Hawaii: 1–800–518–8887
Idaho: 1–800–926–2588
Illinois: 1–800–226–0768
Indiana: 1–800–889–9949
Kansas: 1–800–766–9012
Kentucky: 1–877–524–4718
Louisiana: 1–877–252–2447
Maine: 1–800–452–4694
Maryland: 1–800–402–5231
Massachusetts: 1–800–841–2900
Michigan: 1–888–988–6300
Minnesota: 1–800–657–3739
Mississippi: 1–800–421–2408

Missouri: 1–888–275–5908
Montana: 1–877–543–7669
Nebraska: 1–877–632–5437
Nevada: 1–800–992–0900
New Hampshire: 1–877–464–2447
New Jersey: 1–800–701–0701
New Mexico: 1–800–432–6217
New York: 1–800–698–4543
North Carolina: 1–800–367–2229
North Dakota: 1–800–755–2604
Ohio: 1–800–324–8680
Oklahoma: 1–800–987–7767
Pennsylvania: 1–800–842–2020
Rhode Island: 1–401–462–5300
South Carolina: 1–888–549–0820
South Dakota: 1–800–305–3064
Tennessee: 1–800–669–1851
Texas: 1–800–647–6558
Utah: 1–888–222–2542
Vermont: 1–800–250–8427
Virginia: 1–877–822–6764
Washington: 1–877–543–7669
West Virginia: 1–888–983–2645
Wisconsin: 1–800–441–4576
Wyoming: 1–800–251–1269

REFERENCES

Albrecht, M. N. (1991). Home health care: Reliability and validity testing of a patient classification instrument. *Public Health Nursing, 8,* 124–131.

American Academy of Pediatrics. (2001). *Medicaid and SCHIP income eligibility guidelines for children.* Elk Grove Village, IL: American Academy of Pediatrics.

American Academy of Pediatrics Committee on Children with Disabilities. (1998). Managed care and children with special health care needs: A subject review. *Pediatrics, 102,* 657–660.

American Academy of Pediatrics Committee on Children with Disabilities. (2001). The continued importance of Supplemental Security Income (SSI) for children and adolescents with disabilities. *Pediatrics, 107*(4), 790–793.

American Academy of Pediatrics Reference Committee on Child Health Financing. (2001). Implementation principles and strategies for the State Children's Health Insurance Program. *Pediatrics, 107*(5), 1214–1218.

Amonkar, M., Madharan, S., Rosenbluth, S., Odeding, T., & Simon, K. (2000). Assessing managed care's role in promoting preventive care. *Journal of Community Health, 25*(3), 225–240.

Bandura, A. (1977). *Social learning theory.* Englewood Cliffs, NJ: Prentice-Hall.

Boosfeld, B., & O'Toole, M. (2000). Technology-dependent children: Transition from hospital to home. *Pediatric Nursing, 12*(6), 20–22.

Donabedian, A. (1980). *Explorations in quality assessment and monitoring: The definition of quality and approaches to its assessment.* Ann Arbor, MI: Health Administration Press.

Faulkner, M. S. (1999). Quality of life for persons with developmental disabilities. *Scholarly Inquiry for Nursing Practice, an International Journal, 23*(3), 239.

Fink, M. L. (1993). Managed care is not the answer. *Journal of Health, Politics, Policy and Law, 18*(1), 105–112.

Fleming, J. (1993). *Home health care of technology dependent children.* Unpublished report, University of Kentucky, Lexington.

Frisch, N. C., Dossey, B. M., Guzzetta, C. E., & Quinn, J. A. (2000). *AHNA standards of holistic nursing practice: Guidelines for caring and healing.* Gaithersburg, MD: Aspen.

Glendinning, C., Kirk, S., Guiffrida, A., & Lawton, D. (2000). Technology dependent children in the community: Definitions, numbers and costs. *Child Health Care and Development, 27*(4), 321–334.

Haddad, A. M. (1996). The evolution of high-tech home care. In L. A. Garski (Ed.), *High Tech Home Care Manual* (pp. 1.1–1.8). Gaithersburg, MD: Aspen.

Hernandez, J. A., Offutt, J., & Butterfield, H. J. (1986). The cost of care of the less-than-1000 gm. infant. *Clinical Perinatology, 13*(2), 461–471.

Hobbs, N., Perrin, J. M., & Ireys, H. T. (1993). *Chronically ill children and their families.* San Francisco: Jossey-Bass.

Holdsworth, M. T., Raisch, D. W., Chavez, C. M., Duncan, M. H., Parasuraman, T. V., & Fox, F. M. (1997). Economic impact with home delivery of chemotherapy to pediatric oncology patients. *Annals of Pharmacology, 31*(2), 140–148.

Institute of Medicine. (2000). *Informing the future.* Washington, DC: National Academy of Science.

Kettrick, R. G., & Donar, M. E. (1985). The ventilator dependent child: Medical and social care. *Critical Care: State of the Art, 6*, 1–38.

King, I. M. (1994). Quality of life and goal attainment. *Nursing Science Quarterly, 7*(1), 29–32.

Marshall, P. A. (1990). Cultural influences on perceived quality of life. *Seminars in Oncology Nursing, 6*, 276–284.

Manificat, S., Guilland-Bataille, J. M., & Dazord, A. (1993). Quality of life in children with chronic disease: Review of literature and conceptual aspects. *Pediatrics, 48*, 519–527.

McLaughlin, J. F., & Bjornson, K. F. (1998). Quality of life and developmental disabilities. *Developmental Medicine & Child Neurology, 40,* 435.

Office of Technology Assessment. (1987). Technology-dependent children: Hospital vs. home care—a technical memorandum. Washington, DC: U.S. Government Printing Office.

Parette, H. P., Jr. (1993). High-risk infant case management and assistive technology: Funding and family enabling perspectives. *Maternal-Child Health Nursing Journal, 21,* 53–64.

Pless, I. B. (1974). *Theoretical and practical considerations in the measurement of outcome in chronic childhood illness assessment of outcome.* DHEW Publications No (NIH) 76-877. Washington, DC: U.S. Department of Health, Education and Welfare.

Sisk, J. E., Gorman, S. A., Reisirger, A. J., Glied, S. A., DuMouchel, W. H., & Hynes, M. M. (1996). Evaluation of Medicaid managed care: Satisfaction, access and use. *Journal of the American Medical Association, 276,* 50–55.

Smith, C. (1995). Technology and home care. In J. J. Fitzpatrick & J. S. Stevenson (Eds.), *Annual Review of Nursing Research* (pp. 13, 137–167). New York: Springer.

Smith, C. (1996). Quality of life and caregiving in technological home care. In J. J. Fitzpatrick & J. Norbeck (Eds.), pp. 14, 95–118. New York: Springer.

Task Force on Technology Dependent Children. (1988). *Fostering home and community-based care for technology dependent children.* Washington, DC: U.S. Department of Health and Human Services, U.S. Government Printing Office.

Varricchio, C. (1994). Human and indirect costs of home care. *Nursing Outlook, 42,* 151–157.

Weiner, J. P., & deLissovoy, (1993). Razing a tower of babel: A taxonomy for managed care and health care plans. *Journal of Health, Politics, Policy and Law, 18*(1), 75–103.

Wielawski, I. M. (1998). Rationing medical care: The growing gulf between what's medically available and what's affordable. *Advances—The Robert Wood Johnson Foundation Special Supplement,* Issue 4, 1–7.

Chapter 12

Finding Respite Care and Other Community Resources

Respite care is viewed as an important caregiving resource and an essential part of the overall support that families may need to keep their technology-dependent children at home. Respite was identified as a component of appropriate care and on a scale of 1 to 5 was seen as the number 1 priority (Task Force on Technology Dependent Children, 1988). Breckbill and Carmen (1994) indicate that one home health agency staff identified community needs and developed three pediatric programs to address that need. The programs were case management, a respite program, and a parent education program to prevent child abuse and neglect. They report that the programs strengthened the families and the community this agency serves.

THE CONCEPT OF RESPITE CARE

The respite movement, which started in the 1960s with the concept of deinstitutionalization, developed with the belief that the best place to care for a child with special needs was in the child's home and community. Respite care has been defined as a system of temporary supports for families of developmentally disabled individuals which provide the family with relief. Respite care services may be provided in the home or outside the home in various settings in the community. In addition to providing direct relief, respite care has additional benefits for families (National Information Center for Children and Youth with Disabilities, 1996). The added benefits noted were

- **Relaxation**—Respite gives families peace of mind, helps them relax, and renews their humor and their energy.

- Enjoyment—Respite allows families to enjoy favorite pastimes and pursue new activities.
- Stability—Respite improves the family's ability to cope with daily responsibilities and maintain stability during crises.
- Preservation—Respite helps preserve the family unit and lessens the pressures that might lead to institutionalization, divorce, neglect, and child abuse.
- Involvement—Respite allows families to become involved in community activities and to feel less isolated.
- Time Off—Respite allows families to take that needed vacation, spend time together, and time alone.
- Enrichment—Respite makes it possible for family members to establish individual identities and enrich their growth and development.

The concept of respite as a community service is based on understanding and dealing with family concerns and perceptions of family problem. The concept encompasses the wider social context in which the family lives. Respite services always should be designed to meet the needs of the family. Families' needs will dictate the type of service they should have, as not all families have the same needs. If what is best for a family is not currently available, the information may serve as a means to develop the service in the community. Respite care has gained support at the federal level as a result of the passage of Children's Justice Act (Public Law 99-401) and its amendment, the Children's and Disabilities Temporary Care Reauthorization Act (Public Law 101-127).

RESEARCH ON RESPITE CARE

A variety of approaches to respite care and (for some) the effectiveness of those approaches have been reported in the literature. A few of the more recent ones are noted here. Menezes (2001) examines the development of a children's hospice service. The service provides, for families living in specific areas in England, palliative and respite care in their own homes (community care) backed up by a respite care service in a related hospice. Olsen and Maslim-Prothero (2001) provide the findings of a parent-centered follow-up evaluation using in-depth qualitative interviews of 18 families. The evaluation revealed the sometimes mixed reaction to an innovative nurse-led home-based respite service for families of children under the age of 5 with complex health care needs. The authors explore the diverse ways that respite service can support the need of this client group and the need for flexibility in the kind of service being provided if families' support needs are not met. Neufeld, Query, and Drummond (2001) describe the use of respite service by primary caregivers of children with chronic illness and disabilities, perceptions of actual respite, and barriers to respite and respite care. They found that despite accessing a variety of respite services, the participants perceived limited actual respite from caregiving. A census was taken of families in Northern Ireland who used six types of short-term break services during a 12-month period: (1) hospital-based overnight care, (2) overnight stays in a residential home, (3) domiciliary service in the family home, (4) breaks provided in another family home, (5) residential holidays, and (6) breaks provided through leisure schemes organized after school or during holidays for their child with disabilities. A second study using interviews was done regarding families' usage and preference for each type of service. Variations in parental preference and usage were identified. The information will be used to assist commissioners in developing cost-beneficial short-break services.

The impact of respite care services for families caring for children experiencing emotional and behavioral problems was studied by Bruns and Burchard (2000). Results of a controlled, longitudinal study of the short-term effectiveness of respite care showed that the 33 families who received respite care experienced significantly better outcomes overall than did 28 families on a wait-list comparison group, including fewer incidents of out-of-home placement and greater options about caring for the child.

Cuttell and Gartland (1999) report on a 5-year experience with a hospital-based home care renal nursing service. During the 5-year period, 286 respite care visits were performed for children aged 2 months to 15 years who were on continuous cycling peritoneal dialysis. The parental response to the home care support resulted in a home care nurse being incorporated into the budget. The new nursing post raised issues of professional accountability of home care nurses, of patient confidentiality, and of communication with multidisciplinary team members.

Several authors have mentioned respite care from the perspective of meeting of the complex health or special needs of the child and family (Kendle & Campanale, 2001; Robinson, Jackson, & Townsley, 2001). A critical factor in using respite care services is knowing about them. Some respite services in the community are for specific health problems and may not be available to children who are dependent on technology, while others in the community may be available to them. To access a service, information is essential. Hayes, Cotterill, Sloper, and Flynn (1998) note that the ability of users and their parents or carers to choose services hinges on what they know about them. Their results of a survey of Social Services Department in England suggest that information may not reach all of those who could benefit from respite.

Teschendorf and Vassallo (1984) describe a nursing service pediatric program that was instituted to complement the services of a local under-staffed cerebral palsy center. This creative early intervention program reflects how nursing and physical therapy professionals worked together to educate the parental caregiver and enhance the home care of children and means for respite.

Mausner (1995) describes a family support project that implemented a cost-effective, family-centered approach to the provision of home-based respite care for severely handicapped children who had complex medical needs. Links of families with provider families who learned to care for these children resulted in the provision of respite care for the families who had the children with complex conditions. Weilber (1995) describes project CARE (Children with AIDS Respite Experience) an innovative in-home respite program for children with AIDS at New York Hospital–Cornell University Medical Center. Children are usually taken out of the home so that parent can rest during the respite visit. Strategies to recruit, train, and supervise volunteers along with support and evaluation are presented.

Factors associated with respite care are described by Wherry, Schema, Baltz, and Kelleher (1995). Users and nonusers of respite care of parents with a disabled child were compared. Fifty-four of the 66 families interviewed used respite care services, and 12 families did not. No differences were found in use based on age, number of family members, family income, or needs of the child. Rural responders expressed concern about travel distances.

Weilber (1995) discusses strategies used in an innovative in-home respite care program for caregivers of HIV-positive children. The project provided a minimum of 4 hours weekly of child care for children in the home. The amount of service provided is determined by the minimum time needed by the parent. During respite visit, the volunteers take the child out of the home.

The relationship between stress and coping of parents with a child who is disabled can be considered from a perspective of personal and socio-ecological coping resources. Coping strategies used by parents vary. Beresford (1994) describes both personal and socio-ecological coping resources and the vulnerability of the point when the resources are no longer available. The relationship between coping strategies and adjustment was explored.

Boosfeld and O'Toole (2000) indicate that the primary reason for achieving home care for children who are technology dependent and who have complex and special needs is not to create a hospital in the home, but to achieve safety for the child as simply as possible, with the least disruption to normal family life. Parental caregivers cannot afford to allow their personal concerns to interfere with the professionals who provide their expertise in the care of their children. A study (Patterson, Jernell, Leonard, & Titus, 1994) of 48 mothers and fathers of medically fragile children who were cared for in the home revealed strain for mothers with home care providers. The strain was explained by four variables: more hours of care from the home health aide increased the strain; perceived support from the community reduced the strain; belief in family strengths increased the strain; and better organization reduced the strain. In the discussion, the authors note that for mothers, it was only more help from home health aides caring for their children (in contrast to help with the child from professional nurses or help with housework from a homemaker) that added to the mothers' burden in the parent-professional relationship.

Educators in preparing future professionals to work with families need to help students identify early what are the personal dynamics that creates feelings of strain or burden in professional-parent relationships. Health professionals could benefit from research that more fully would delineate the relationship between parents and professionals. In discussing the promotion of family adaptation to home care of children who are technology dependent, Smith (1991) concludes that families who are caring for these children at home not only have technical skills to learn, provide, and include in the activities of their daily lives but also have to adjust to the psychosocial factors of home care and to the different parenting skills a special needs child requires. The professionals have a responsibility to help them adapt to the unique situation in which they find themselves.

Watson, Townsley, and Abbott (2002) describe an ongoing research study that is exploring the impact of multiagency work on children with complex needs that typically require technical and/or medical equipment in the home and on their families. Valkenier, Hayes, and McElheran (2002) examine mothers' experiences of receiving in-home nursing respite care for their children with medically fragile and complex conditions. Their findings contribute to nursing knowledge about meeting in-home respite needs of mothers of children with complex medical conditions. Implications for nursing include how to better support maternal coping, decrease uncertainty, and foster more effective relationships with the mothers of these children.

Providing care for children with special care needs is a challenge. A 10-year action plan to achieve community-based service system which included respite services for these children and their families is highlighted in Pediatric Nursing (2001). Using a Grounded Theory Methodology, Kirk (2001) conducted a study to assess the transfer of responsibility from professionals to parents of children who were involved in providing highly technical care to their children. In-depth interviews were done with 23 mothers, 10 fathers, and 44 professionals to gain insight into the experience of caring for children at home with complex health care needs.

Kirk concludes that (1) parental choice was constrained initially by parents' feelings of obligation and by the lack of community services, and (2) nurses are ideally placed to play the central role not only in ensuring that role negotiation and discussion actually occur in practice but also in asserting the need for appropriate community support services for families.

FINDING RESPITE SERVICES

Nurses helping families with the home care of children who are technology dependent will likely be involved in assisting them with the selection of respite services that best meet their needs. Following are some suggestions in providing assistance.

1. Does the family need short-term, long-term, or both types of service? Will the service be in the home or at the service facility?
2. What agency in the community can provide the service needed?
3. What is the cost? Will insurance, Medicaid, or some other form of payment be made to the provider of the service?
4. What is the procedure for use of the service?
5. Information about the quality of the service such as training of personnel, safety of service, policies of service, etc. should be obtained.

Recognition that parents may have fears about using respite and other services in the community is important. Borfittz-Mescon (1998) indicates that the anxiety that parents may have resulting from normal and real concerns or fears can in fact cause parents to believe that respite service is just not worth it. Helping the parents become comfortable with the decision to use respite or other services in the community is important for their well-being and peace of mind.

Several agencies and organizations in the community have information on family support services. Some are identified below that may be useful for families with children who are technology dependent.

ARCH National Resource Center for Crisis Nurseries and Respite Care Services
Chapel Hill Training Outreach Project, 800 Eastowne Drive, Suite 105, Chapel Hill, NC 27514; Phone: 1–800–773–5433.
The Center's mission is to provide support to service providers through training, technical assistance, evaluation and research. It operates the National Respite Locator Service, whose mission is to help parents locate respite care services in their area.

American Association of University Affiliated Programs (AAUAP)
8630 Fenton Street, Suite 410, Silver Spring, MD 20910; Phone: 1–301–588–8252.
AAUAP represents the national network of University Affiliated Programs (UAPs) in the United States. The UAPs provide interdisciplinary training for professionals and paraprofessionals and offer programs and services for children with disabilities and their families.

National Clearinghouse on Family Support and Children's Mental Health
Portland State University, P.O. 751, Portland, OR 97207–0751; Phone: 1–800–628–1696.
The Center provides research and training and disseminates information relative to serious emotional disorders and family support issues.

Association for the Care of Children's Health (ACCH)
7910 Woodmont Avenue, Suite 300, Bethesda, MD; Phone: 1–800–808–2224.

Association for Persons with Severe Handicaps
29 West Susquehanna Avenue, Suite 210, Baltimore, MD 21204; Phone: 1–410–828–8274.

Beach Center on Families and Disability
University of Kansas, 3111 Haworth Hall, Lawrence, KS 66045; Phone: 1–913–864–7600.
The Center provides information about families with members who

have disabilities and provides links to parent-to-parent support through state and local chapters.

SECURITY ISSUES

The health care environment must be safe for the children, their families, and the professionals who serve them in their homes and community service agencies. Considering that home health care is a major component of an integrated health care system, security issues for the patient and the family are important as well as for the professional caregiver.

For Professionals

Prescreening patients before visit (clear instructions). Call before scheduled visit. If home is in an area known for high crime or drugs, health visitor should schedule the visit as early in the day as possible, and on the way to the home should call the local police and let them know they are going to the area and will call them from the home. Staff member should be provided with a cellular phone.

Key Points

- There are both internal and external aspects of home health care security;
- Agencies interviewing applicants for home health care positions should do thorough criminal history background checks;
- Home health care patients should be prescreened to see if they may be violent;
- Staff should be able to adjust the time-of-day or night that visits are made to assist in their protection; and
- Staff must be taught security techniques to use while on the road, on the street and in the home.

REFERENCES

Beresford, B. A. (1994). Resources and strategies: How parents cope with the care of a disabled child. *Journal of Child Psychology Psychiatry*, 35(1), 171–209.

Bond, N., Phillips, P., & Rollins, J. A. (1994). Family centered care at home for families with children who are technology dependent. *Pediatric Nursing, 20*(2), 123–130.

Boosfeld, B., & O'Toole, M. (2000). Technology-dependent children: Transition from hospital to home. *Pediatric Nursing, 12*(6), 20–22.

Borfittz-Mescon, J. (1998). Parent written care plans: Instructions for the respite setting. *The Exceptional Parent, 18*(3), 20–25.

Breckbill, J., & Carmen, S. (1994). Support for families with special needs. *Caring, 13*(12), 42–46.

Bruns, E., & Burchard, J. D. (2000). Impact of respite care services for families with children experiencing emotional and behavioral problems. *Children's Services: Social Policy, Research and Practice, 3*(1), 39–61.

Camp, C. J., Doherty, K., Moody-Thomas, S., & Denney, N. W. (1989). Practical problem-solving in adults: A comparison of problem types and scoring methods. In J. D. Sinnett (Ed.), *Everyday problem-solving: Theory and applications* (pp. 211–228). New York: Praeger.

Cuttell, K., & Gartland, C. (1999). Five years' experience of a hospital-based home-care renal nursing service. *Advances in Peritoneal Dialysis—Conference on Peritoneal Dialysis, 15,* 258–261.

DeKvok, M., & Gerris, J. N. (1992). Parental reasoning complexity, social class and childrearing behaviors. *Journal of Marriage and the Family, 54,* 675–685.

Feeg, V. D. (2001). Understanding children with special care needs: A national pediatric challenge. *Pediatric Nursing, 27*(4), 342.

Hayes, L., Cotterill, L., Sloper, P., & Flynn, M. (1998). Finding out about and accessing respite (short-term breaks). *British Journal of Learning Disabilities, 24*(3), 115–118.

Holden, G. W. (1988). Adult's thinking about a child-rearing problem: Effects of experience parental status, and gender. *Child Development, 59,* 1623–1632.

Kendle, J., & Campanale, R. (2001). A pediatric learning experience: Respite care for families with children with special needs. *Nurse Educator, 26*(2), 95–98.

Kirk, S. (1999). Focus on children's nursing: Caring for technology dependent children at home. *British Journal of Community Nursing, 4*(8), 390–394.

Kirk, S. (2001). Negotiating lay and professional roles in the care of children with complex health care needs. *Journal of Advanced Nursing, 34*(5), 593–602.

Mausner, S. (1995). Families helping families: An innovative approach to the provision of respite care for families of children with complex medical needs. *Social Work in Health Care, 21*(1), 95–106.

McGonigel, M., Kaufmann, R., & Johnson, B. (Eds.). (1991). *Guidelines and recommended practices for individualized family service plan* (2nd ed.). Bethesda, MD: Association for the Care of Children's Health.

Menezes, A. (2001). Reflections on the development of CHASE Children's Hospice Service. *Journal of Child Health Care, 5*(3), 123–125.

National Information Center for Children and Youth with Disabilities. (1996). Briefing Paper Respite Care. Washington, DC.

Neufeld, S. M., Query, B., & Drummond, J. E. (2001). Respite care users who have children with chronic conditions: Are they getting a break? *Journal of Pediatric Nursing, 16*(4), 234–244.

O'Brien, M. E. (2001). Living in a house of cards: Family experiences with long term childhood technology dependence. *Journal of Pediatric Nursing, 16*(1), 13–22.

Olsen, R., & Maslim-Prothero, P. (2001). Dilemmas in the provision of own home respite support for parents of young children with complex health care needs: Evidence from an evaluation. *Journal of Advanced Nursing, 34*(5), 603–610.

Patterson, J. M., Jernell, M. A., Leonard, B. J., & Titus, J. C. (1994). Caring for medically fragile children at home: The parent-professional relationship. *Journal of Pediatric Nursing, 9*(2), 98–106.

Robinson, C., Jackson, P., & Townsley, R. (2001). Short breaks for families caring for a disabled child with complex needs. *Child and Family Social Work, 6*(1), 67–75.

Rubin, K. H., Mills, R. S. L., & Rose-Krasnor, L. (1989). Maternal beliefs and children's competence. In B. H. Schneider, G. Ajile, J. Nadel, & R. P. Weissberg (Eds.), *Social competence in development perspective* (pp. 313–331). Boston: Kluwer Academic Publishers.

Sells, D. H., Jr. (2000). *Security in the health care environment.* Gaithersburg, MD: Aspen.

Smith, J. (1991). Promoting family adaptation to the at home care of the technology dependent child. *Issues in Comprehensive Pediatric Nursing, 14,* 249–258.

Task Force on Technology Dependent Children. (1988). Fostering home and community-based care for technology-dependent children. Report to Congress. Washington, DC: U.S. Government Printing Office.

Teschendorf, B., & Vassallo, D. (1984). Home care pediatric early intervention pays off. *Clinical Management, 4*(1), 34–37.

Valkenier, B. J., Hayes, V. E., & McElheran, P. J. (2002). Mothers' perspectives on an in-home respite service: Coping and control. *Canadian Journal of Nursing Research, 34*(1), 87–109.

Watson, D., Townsley, R., & Abbott, D. (2002). Exploring multi-agency working in services to disabled children with complex health care needs and their families. *Journal of Clinical Nursing, 11*(3), 367–375.

Weilber, J. (1995). Respite care for HIV-affected families. *Social Work in Health Care, 21*(1), 55–67.

Wherry, J. N., Schema, S. J., Baltz, T., & Kelleher, K. (1995). Factors associated with respite care used by families with a child with disabilities. *Journal of Child and Family Studies, 4*(4), 419–428.

Chapter 13

Advocating for Patients and Families: A Policy Perspective

From a policy perspective, it is interesting to note that in spite of the fact that the United States spends more money per person on its blended public-private health care system than any other nation in the world, it ranks 37th in the world on how well it prevents illness and serves the poor and minorities (Neergaard, 2000). The families of technology-dependent children often have difficulty negotiating the health care system. This chapter describes how nurses can better advocate for families.

UNDERSTANDING MANAGED CARE

Managed care appears to be the primary system designed to offer health care in this society. Ninety-one percent of employees with health insurance were enrolled in managed care plans in 1999 (Institute of Medicine, 2000). There are pros and cons about managed health care systems. Fleming (1993) notes that most of the over 800 caregivers in a study of children who were technology dependent and receiving home care were primarily white and middle class. It is interesting, too, that few resided in rural areas. Most resided in a suburban area or the city (see Table 13.1). Could rationing of health care be one of the reasons for this? Services for individuals who live in rural areas may not be as readily available as they are for those who reside in urban areas. With the emphasis on cutting costs and physicians having to justify the use of expensive procedures, perhaps the poorer individuals in society, many of whom are from ethnic/racial groups that are not white, are those who do not have health insurance. Wielawski (1998) notes that there are many forms of rationing. She notes that managed care and other changes in the health care system have reduced surplus

TABLE 13.1　Caregivers Residence

Residence	N	%
Rural area—farm	10	1.2
Rural area—non-farm	61	7.2
Small town	197	23.2
Suburb	251	29.6
City	325	38.3
Does not know	1	0.1
Unidentified	3	0.3

money that used to be available to cover free care for the poor. It seems that if families who care for children in their home don't have insurance and/or other means to help provide care in their homes, home care is not a viable alternative.

Amonkar, Madharan, Rosenbluth, Odeding, and Simon (2000) note that the current trend of managed care health systems opens the door to more effective control of chronic diseases through preventive care. Using a mailed questionnaire, a national sample of 1,200 directors associated with preventive care in a managed care organization (MCO) were surveyed. They found that case management was perceived by respondent MCOs to be the most effective and important strategy in ensuring appropriate utilization of preventive services, followed by use of prospective utilization review programs. Smucker (2001) notes that providing care to children with special health care needs within a managed care environment presents special challenges for providers and parents. Children and families in managed care programs may experience limited access to specialized care and services along with decreased fragmentation inherent in fee-for-service care. Pediatric nurse practitioners can play a significant role in ensuring that children receive the most appropriate care.

The outcome of care is relevant. If managed care is to survive, consumers must believe that the health care services they receive are quality services. Professionals providing health care services to children who are technology dependent and cared for in their homes will have to be accountable as they will be judged by consumers and purchasers of health care. Patient/ consumer satisfaction is gaining as an important outcome in health care delivery as the health care system continues the managed care approach. (Donabedian, 1980; Sisk et al., 1996).

The trend toward holding health care providers more accountable is increasing in all practice settings. The importance of improving communication to patients, maintaining competence, and using innovative approaches to transform the care of children who are technology dependent and being cared for in their homes cannot be overstated. Quality report cards are being used to evaluate care and consumer's choices. Trying to determine the best performing hospitals, physicians, nurses, health plans, and so on is likely to continue and may result in improved services. Best-practices guidelines and evidence-based practices are other approaches being implemented in health care delivery. All of these approaches are designed for performance improvement in health care organizations, which is positive. Managed care has resulted in changes in the health care environment. Outcomes and patient satisfaction have resulted in the evaluation of care that health practitioners provide.

ADVOCATING FOR APPROPRIATE CARE

Chapman and Chapman (1975) use three dimensions to classify advocacy (see Table 13.2). The potential use of their framework to identify and classify the advocacy needs of children who are technology dependent may be of value to health care providers.

The recognition of advocacy of nursing seems particularly relevant. This recognition does not minimize the services of other professionals but views the problem from a perspective that recognizes the complexity or at least how involved providing home care for technology-dependent children may be. Further, the nurse's role is one of a constant contact person and a potential helper to the family in coordinating other services. Attention to the quality of nursing care is very pertinent. Implications for changes in the curriculum of students in nursing programs may be indicated. The type of nurse or paraprofessional needed may depend on the nature and complexity of the child's problem and the family dynamics. It seems easy to measure specific technical skills but more difficult to measure other skills that may be provided by nurses.

Advocacy for children who are technology dependent is reflected in the three components identified by the Task Force on Technology Dependent Children (1988): case management, respite care, and developmental/education services. Each of these components are seen as essential to appropriate care. With some modification, appropriate care as delineated by the task force seems to still be relevant and appropriate. The description of appropriate care below has been adapted from the task force components:

TABLE 13.2   Advocacy Classifications

Evaluation Dimensions	Definitions of Evaluative Dimensions

I. Life saving
    A. Primary
	I. Prevention of imminent death
	    A. Unanticipated emergency
	    B. Emergencies secondary to such states as disease and trauma

II. Life sustaining
 	
    A. Primary
 	
    B. Secondary
 	
    C. Tertiary
	II. Maintenance of health and prevention of disability complications in living
	    A. Maintenance of good health through prevention of disease, injury, and developmental deviations
	    B. Prevention of disease or disabling complications in living from disease, illness, or developmental deviations
	    C. Prevention of disabling complications in dying (e.g., physical and emotional suffering)

III. Life enhancing
 	
    A. Primary
 	
    B. Secondary
 	
    C. Tertiary
	III. Maintenance, restoration, or development of a person's relationship with the world such that the person feels emotional well-being, social productive, and self-satisfied
	    A. Prevention of disabling complications in interpersonal relationships from social-emotional problems in living
	    B. Prevention of interpersonal problems in living secondary to effects of disease, drugs, injury, or developmental deviation
	    C. Prevention of dehumanizing residential care giving through establishment of humanistic helping goals

Appropriate Care

1. Appropriate care is

- the technical and psychosocial care necessary to effectively operate devices and perform services needed to sustain life and avoid further disability
- professional training and monitoring of caregivers in providing technical, nursing, and personal care

- support services necessary to enable caregivers to provide continuous, consistent and competent care

2. Appropriate care is care that
    - does not attempt to duplicate an institutional setting
    - is less costly than institutional care in terms of some direct costs in the short term, but may be costly in terms of indirect costs
    - is planned by a formal managed care program to meet specific needs of individual children and their families
    - includes a separate quality of care system to ensure the program works effectively

3. Appropriate care is
    - services and equipment necessary to sustain life in the home or community setting
    - services and equipment that are safe, readily available, reliable, of good quality, and user-friendly to caregivers
    - at least equal in quality to the care provided in the institution and should be cost-effective

4. Appropriate care is diagnosis- and severity-specific medical care provided to an individual with a diagnosed illness or condition that would be recognized as accepted medical practice by most health care providers.

5. Appropriate care is a comprehensive set of individual, family, and community-oriented services. Individual services might include surgical, medical, nursing, case management, early identification and screening, and counseling. Family services might include affordable health insurance, transportation, respite care, housing adaptation, parent-to-parent support, and parent training. Community services might include public advocacy, quality assurance, interagency coordination, and support services not covered by health insurance.

6. Appropriate care is health care of the level and frequency that will cause the patient's condition to stabilize or improve while reducing the incidence of adverse outcomes from the disease process or the treatment itself.

7. Appropriate care is the type and amount of specialized personal care required by technology-dependent children to
    - maintain life support

- provide an environment conducive to growth and emotional development
- stimulate learning
- provide the least restrictive setting

ADVOCACY SOURCES

Advocacy for families caring for these special needs children is vital to ensuring that their physical, emotional, social, and health care needs are met. Some recommended resources for families follow.

Families

KDWB Variety Family Center
University of Minnesota Gateway, 200 Oak Street SE, Suite 160, Minneapolis, MN 55455–2002; Phone: 1–612–626–2401; Web sites: www.peds. umn.edu/peds-adol/; www.cyfc.umn.edu/NRL/.

This center focuses on children and adolescents with disabilities and chronic illnesses and their families and includes clinical services, academic pediatrics, a family resource center, and a walk-in center where families can obtain materials related to their child's disability or chronic condition. Clinical services available at the center include the STAR Center, behavioral pediatrics, U Special Kids, pediatric psychology, and general pediatrics. The center also has a database.

The Family Village
The Waisman Center, University of Wisconsin-Madison, 1500 Highland Avenue, Madison, WI 53705–2280; E-mail: familyvillage@waisman. wisc.edu; Web site: www.familyvillage.isc.edu/.

The Family Village provides access to a great deal of information for parents and professionals. The Web site has links to a large number of other sites, including alternative treatments, pharmaceutical sources, and recreation and leisure activities.

National Information Center for Children and Youth with Disabilities
P.O. Box 1492, Washington, DC 20013; Voice/TDD: 1–800–695–0285; 1–202–884–8200; Fax: 1–202–884–8441; E-mail: nichcy@aed.org; Web site: www.nichcy.org.

This center provides a wide variety of information to parents and professionals and offers referrals to other organizations.

Parent Advocacy Coalition for Educational Rights (PACER) Center
4826 Chicago Avenue South, Minneapolis; MN 55417–1098; Phone: 1–612–827–2966; 1–800–537–2237 (in Minnesota); 1–612–827–7770 (TDD); Fax: 1–612–827–3065; 1–800–848–4912; Web site: www.pacer. org.
PACER provides educational and training to help parents understand the special education laws and to obtain appropriate school programs for their children. It also offers information on child abuse prevention, newsletters, booklets, extensive written materials, and videotapes.

Family Voices National Office
P.O. Box 769, Algodones, NM 87001: Phone 1–888–835–5669; 1–505–867–2368; Fax: 1–505–867–6517; E-mail: kidshealth@familyvoices.org; Web site: www.familyvoices.org.
This parent organization provides advocacy and support, publishes a bimonthly newsletter, and has chapters in each state.

Federation for Children with Special Needs
1135 Tremont Street, Suite 420, Boston, MA 02120; Phone: 1–617–236–7210; 1–800–331–0688 (toll-free in Massachusetts only); Fax: 1–617–572–2094; E-mail: fcsninfo@fcsn.org; Web site: www.fcsn.org.
This center for parents and parent groups offers links to parent training centers in different states.

National Parent to Parent Support and Information System Inc. (NPPSIS)
P.O. Box 907, Blue Ridge, GA 30513; Phone: 1–800–651–1151 (for parents); 1–706–374–6250 (Head Start) (TDD available); Fax: 1–706–374–3826; E-mail: nppsis@ellijay.com; Web site: www.nppsis.org.
This organizations provides information and links to other families for support.

Siblings

The Sibling Support Project
Children's Hospital and Regional Medical Center, P.O. Box 5371, CL–09, Seattle, WA 98105–0371; Phone: 1–206–527–5712; Fax: 1–206–527–5705; E-mail: dmeyer@cmc.org; Web site: www.chmc.org/departmt/sibsupp/.

This national program is dedicated to the interests of brothers and sisters of people with special health and developmental needs. It provides a national directory of sibling workshops and publishes a quarterly newsletter.

Fathers

The Fathers Network
Kindering Center, 16120 N.E. Eighth Street, Bellevue, WA 98008–3937; Phone: 1–206–747–4004, extension 218; 1–206–284–2859; Fax: 1–206–747–1069; 1–206–284–9664; E-mail: Jmay@fathersnetwork.org; Web site: www.fathersnetwork.org.

This advocacy organization for fathers of children with disabilities provides assistance with the development of fathers' groups and publishes a quarterly newsletter.

Policy Issues

The Sullivan v. Zebley Case
This landmark case is important to the home care of children who are technology dependent because these children can now be assessed using the criteria that resulted from the Supreme Court's ruling on the case. Parents caring for these children at home can receive Supplemental Security Income that can help defray expenses of care.

Provisions for benefits for disabled children were a part of the 1972 legislation that established the Supplemental Security Income (SSI) program, which became operational in 1974. The Social Security Administration (SSA) determined that a child was not disabled if the child's impairment did not meet or was not equivalent to one of the listings of impairments that were used to make the determination. No additional evaluation steps for children were provided.

On February 20, 1990, the Supreme Court, in the case of *Sullivan v. Zebley*, decided that the SSA's regulations implementing the law for evaluating disability in children did not adequately reflect congressional intent. The court held that the "listings-only" approach SSA had used to evaluate the disabilities of children did not carry out the "comparable severity" standard in the law, in that the listings were set at a level of severity stricter than the level at which an adult worker can be found disabled and SSA's former policies did not provide for an assessment of overall functional impairment. The court concluded that although the vocational analysis used in adult claims is inapplicable to childhood cases, this does not mean that a functional analysis cannot be applied to them. The SSA read the Supreme Court's decision as holding that children are entitled to an "individualized functional assessment" as a part of the SSA's disability determination process.

The Department of Health and Human Services and the SSA announced on March 23, 1990, that experts in child development and childhood disability representing a wide range of ages were asked to meet with SSA representatives and assist in devising new regulations by supplying input based on their individual expertise. Officials from the SSA and the experts met April 16 and 17, May 3, 4, and 5, and June 28 and 29, 1990. The meetings were open to the public. Other people and advocacy groups were asked for their input as the revision of the rules proceeded. Advice and comments from regional offices were also solicited. The final regulations developed replaced the SSA's prior rules for deciding disability in childhood cases under SSI. As required by the Supreme Court's ruling in *Zebley*, the revised regulations accord each child whose impairment(s) does not medically meet or equal a listing an opportunity to receive an individual assessment of his or her functioning.

Several caregivers of children who were technology dependent had been turned down for SSI benefits prior to this ruling. Many of these children can now obtain these funds. See Chapter 11 for more information on this program and the State Children's Health Insurance Program Plan (SCHIP), which is the most recent significant legislated program on behalf of children.

CONCLUSION

Advocacy by parents and health professionals on behalf of technology-dependent children is a challenge as there are struggles and rewards in caring for a child who is dependent on technology. These children have the same developmental needs as do all children. The achievement of their developmental tasks may in some instances be more difficult. Cohen (1999) notes that the growth of home and community-based care for technology-dependent children is the result of a complex and continuously evolving matrix of medical, social, economic, and technological trends. She further notes the transition process to home and community-based care, however, is not well understood. Roberts (2001) notes that technology's development and application threaten to outpace systems of service delivery. Advocacy is essential to ensure that effective and efficient service is provided to children who rely on medical technology as medical know-how grows more sophisticated. Harrigan, Ratliffe, Patrinos, and Tse (2002) generated a model to improve quality of care and cost effectiveness for medically fragile children. Their review of literature and recommendations for future research consider the sources of stress for families, home care professionals, respite care, financial concerns, and limited community resources. Brannan (2001) examined the relationship between decision-making and family health. This investigator found a positive relationship between decision self-efficacy and family health. Regression analysis supported the hypothesis that family health is significantly influenced by the amount of decisional conflict and decision self-efficacy experienced by parents. As the number of technology-dependent children increases and the diversity of families and communities providing care for them expands, so does the need for research-based models of care that include advocacy, from which to continue developing knowledge and appropriate services.

REFERENCES

Amonkar, M., Madharan, S., Rosenbluth, S., Odeding, T., & Simon, K. (2000). Assessing managed care's role in promoting preventive care. *Journal of Community Health*, 25(3), 225–240.

Bandura, A. (1977). *Social learning theory*. Englewood Cliffs, NJ: Prentice-Hall.

Brannan, J. (2001). Decision-making and health in families with medically fragile children. Doctoral dissertation, University of Missouri, St. Louis.

Chapman, J., & Chapman, H. (1975). *Behavior and health care: A humanistic helping process*. St. Louis, MO: C. V. Mosby.

Cohen, M. (1999). The technology dependent child and the socially marginalized family: A provisional framework. *Qualitative Health Research*, 9(5), 654–667.

Donabedian, A. (1980). *Explorations in quality assessment and monitoring: The definition of quality and approaches to its assessment*. Ann Arbor, MI: Health Administration Press.

Faulkner, M. S. (1999). Quality of life for persons with developmental disabilities. *Scholarly Inquiry for Nursing Practice, an International Journal*, 23(3), 239.

Fink, M. L. (1993). Managed care is not the answer. *Journal of Health, Politics, Policy and Law*, 18(1), 105–112.

Fleming, J. (1993). *Home health care of technology dependent children*. Unpublished report, University of Kentucky, Lexington.

Frisch, N. C., Dossey, B. M., Guzzetta, C. E., & Quinn, J. A. (2000). *AHNA standards of holistic nursing practice: Guidelines for caring and healing*. Gaithersburg, MD: Aspen.

Harrigan, R. C., Ratliffe, C., Patrinos, M. E., & Tse, A. (2002). Medically fragile children: An integrative review of the literature and recommendations for future research. *Issues in Comprehensive Pediatric Nursing, 25*(1), 1–22.

Institute of Medicine. (2000). Informing the future. Changing the Health Care Delivery System (pp. 17–23). *Critical Issues in Health.* Washington, DC: National Academy of Science.

King, I. M. (1994). Quality of life and goal attainment. *Nursing Science Quarterly, 7*(1), 29–32.

Marshall, P. A. (1990). Cultural influences on perceived quality of life. *Seminars in Oncology Nursing, 6,* 276–284.

Manificat, S., Guilland-Bataille, J. M., & Dazord, A. (1993). Quality of life in children with chronic disease: Review of literature and conceptual aspects. *Pediatrics, 48,* 519–527.

McLaughlin, J. F., & Bjornson, K. F. (1998). Quality of life and developmental disabilities. *Developmental Medicine & Child Neurology, 40,* 435.

Neergaard, L. (2000, June 21). U.S. ranks 37th in quality of health care. *Lexington Herald-Leader.*

Roberts, G. (2001). Supporting children with serious health care needs: Analyzing the costs and benefits. *Evaluation and the Health Professions, 24*(1), 72–83.

Sisk, J. E., Gorman, S. A., Reisirger, A. J., Glied, S. A., DuMouchel, W. H., & Hynes, M. M. (1996). Evaluation of Medicaid managed care: Satisfaction, access and use. *Journal of the American Medical Association, 276,* 50–55.

Smucker, J. M. R. (2001). Managed care and children with special health care needs. *Journal of Pediatric Health Care, 15*(1), 3–9.

Task Force on Technology Dependent Children. (1988). *Fostering home and community-based care for technology dependent children.* Washington, DC: U.S. Department of Health and Human Services, U.S. Government Printing Office.

Weiner, J. P., & deLissovoy, (1993). Razing a tower of babel: A taxonomy for managed care and health care plans. *Journal of Health, Politics, Policy and Law, 18*(1), 75–103.

Wielawski, I. M. (1998). Rationing medical care: The growing gulf between what's medically available and what's affordable. *Advances—The Robert Wood Johnson Foundation Special Supplement,* Issue 4, 1–7.

Appendices

Appendix A

Best Practices: ANA Standards of Home Health Care

Where should we look to determine the best practices in nursing care of children who are technology dependent and cared for in their home? Should we consider tradition, experience, advice of colleagues, textbooks, institutional policy, and expert opinion, or shall we focus primarily on research? Evidence-based practice is being touted as the relevant and desirable approach to practice today. What is evidence and why is it important? Is it anecdotal accounts, case studies, expert opinion, or findings from a single research study or several research studies? Today, evidence delineates practice and dictates what it should be. It may help with accreditation standards and decrease costs. It may improve the health and well-being of patients and decrease variability among clinicians and practice sites. Standardization of care may result and costs may be reduced. Best practices require a search of reports of applicable research that has been critically evaluated.

Three basic categories are thought to enter into decision-making. They are (1) evidence (patient data, basic clinical and epidemiology research and systematic reviews), (2) patient/health care provider factors such as cultural beliefs, ethnicity, personal values, experience, education and ethics, and (3) constraints (formal policies, laws, community standards, time, and reimbursements). Knowledge and ethics are important in making clinical decisions. Sound clinical judgment, reasoning, and decision-making, based on evidence from assessments, make up the foundation of best practice in the care of the children who are technology dependent and cared for at home and their families.

Guidelines for clinical practice in caring for children who are technology dependent and cared for in their home are based to some extent on the reviews of scientific literature, some of which is in Chapter 2 and other chapters of this book. However, several approaches may be considered in determining best practices. Systematic reviews are being used to establish evidence-based practice. A systematic review is a scientific investigation. Results from several research studies are synthesized by using an approach that limits bias and error. A caution about the concept of evidence-based practice that clinicians need to recognize is that systematic reviews cannot be relied on solely. Not all outcomes that may be relevant are measured in many studies. Systematic reviews are an important tool, which can be used to help make practice decision. The emphasis on scientific evidence is increasing and may be tied to quality of care. The expectation seems to be growing for more nurses producing and using evidence from research in the delivery of care.

The American Nurses Association (ANA) in 1986 published the Standards of Home Health Nursing Practice. In 1992, the Scope of Practice document for home health nurses complemented the 1986 standards. In 1999 the Association published the Scope and Standards of Home Health Nursing Practice. It provides a template for performance of professional nurses as well as consumers, payers, and policy makers (American Nurses Association, 1999). The Standards of Care delineated by the Association in the Scope and Standards of Home Health Nursing Practice have been adapted here for home care of children who are technology dependent and their family as follows:

STANDARDS OF CARE

Adapted for home care of children who are technology dependent and their families.

Standard I. Assessment

The home health nurse collects information from the family caregiver and the health data for the child who is technology dependent.

Measurement Criteria

1. Data collection involves the child, family, community, and other health care practitioners, as appropriate.

2. The priority of data collection is determined by the child's immediate condition or needs.
3. Pertinent data are collected using appropriate assessment techniques and valid and reliable instruments.
4. Relevant data are documented in a retrievable form.
5. Integrity of the data is confirmed by multiple sources and used in a confidential manner.
6. The data collection process is systematic, ongoing, and comprehensive to the child and his/her family's needs and systems' responses.

Standard II. Diagnosis

The home health nurse analyzes the assessment data in determining diagnoses.

Measurement Criteria

1. Diagnoses are derived from the assessment data.
2. Diagnoses are validated with the physician, the child, family, and other health care practitioners when possible and appropriate.
3. Diagnoses are documented in a manner that facilitates the determination of expected outcomes and plan of care.
4. Diagnoses include condition-specific, health promotion, and disease prevention aspects.

Standard III. Outcome Identification

The home health nurse identifies expected outcomes to the child and child's development and environment.

Measurement Criteria

1. Outcomes are derived from the assessment and diagnoses at two or more points in time.
2. Outcomes are identified as consistent with scientific evidence.
3. Outcomes are mutually formulated with client, family, physician, and other health care practitioners when possible and appropriate.
4. Outcomes are culturally appropriate and realistic in relation to the client's present and potential capabilities.

5. Outcomes are attainable in relation to the resources coordinated for the client.
6. Outcomes include a time estimate for attainment.
7. Outcomes provide direction for continuity of care.
8. Outcomes are documented and measurable.

Standard IV. Planning

The home health nurse develops a plan of care that prescribes intervention to attain expected outcomes.

Measurement Criteria

1. The plan is customized for the child (e.g., age appropriate, culturally sensitive) and the client's condition, needs, and potential.
2. The plan is developed with the family, caregiver, child, physician, and other health care practitioners as appropriate.
3. The plan proposes alternatives for continuity of care along the health care continuum.
4. The plan reflects contemporary resources and acknowledges the cost factor of care within the benefit coverage or other resources.
5. The plan reflects evidence-based nursing practice.
6. The plan provides for continuity of care.
7. Priorities for care are established consistent with the family caregiver and child's desires, benefit package, payer desires, and contemporary evidence.
8. The plan is documented.
9. The plan is sensitive to the changing nature of the child and family needs.

Standard V. Implementation

The home health nurse implements the interventions identified in the plan of care.

Measurement Criteria

1. Interventions are consistent with the established plan of care.
2. Interventions are implemented in a safe, timely, and appropriate manner.

3. Interventions are documented.
4. Interventions are implemented in accordance with the caregiver and child's knowledge as appropriate.

Standard VI. Evaluation

The home health nurse evaluates the child and the family's progress toward attainment of outcomes.

Measurement Criteria

1. Evaluation is systematic, ongoing, and criterion-based.
2. The child, family, and other health care practitioners are involved in the evaluation process as appropriate.
3. Ongoing assessment data are used to revise diagnoses, expected goals, the plan of care, and interventions as needed.
4. Revisions in diagnoses, expected goals, and the plan of care are documented.
5. The effectiveness of interventions is evaluated in relation to outcomes.
6. The client's responses to interventions are documented.
7. Evaluation activities measure efficiency, effectiveness, costs, and consistency with client needs and developing scientific evidence.
8. The practitioner documents the child's and family's outcomes in a manner consistent with reporting requirements.

Standards of professional performance are delineated in the Scope and Standards of Home Health Nursing Practice (American Nurses Association, 1999) and covers standards of quality of care, performance appraisal, education, collegiality, ethics, collaboration, research, and resource utilization. Nurses and health care agencies involved in home health nursing practice are encouraged to purchase the publication from the American Nurses Association. The standards consider the changing nature of home health clients, health care delivery, financing and nursing practice.

As health care delivery changes and as consumers respond to the Patient Bill of Rights, this author believes standards of care will become more of a part of health care professionals' concerns as they deliver care. Nurses who are involved in providing care to children and their families, conducting research, or educating future nurses and who belong to different professional organizations will likely work together in developing and enhancing standards based on evidence that will ensure that the highest quality of care is provided to children and their families. The standards will be such that they represent the best practices for all children, including those who are technology dependent and cared for in their homes.

REFERENCE

American Nurses Association. (1999). *Standards of home health practice.* Washington, DC: American Nurses Publishing.

Appendix B

The Rewards of Participating in Nursing Research: A Collaborator's Perspective

Nora F. Steele

Technology-assisted youth and their families have been the focus of a variety of public and private initiatives since the early 1980s. There have, however, been substantial limitations identified when nurses have considered the practical implications of position papers, research projects, and the large number of small studies. As a clinical nurse specialist working with this population, I found it problematic to plan care based on intuition, experience, and results of studies with divergent populations, rather than generalizable research findings. I strongly supported the need for a national nursing study to examine needs of technology-assisted youth when I learned of the possibility of such a study at the American Nurses' Association (ANA) convention in 1984.

The chronology described here was initially written to document nuances of the High Tech Home Care for Children with Chronic Health Conditions study at one site for the principal investigator. The purpose of this paper is to share a collaborators/co-investigators perspective of a large research project and to demonstrate how research participation can be incorporated into clinical activities, larger populations can be accessed, and validity concerns can be minimized. It may take a long time to plan and implement a multisite, collaborative research project, but the time commitment from individual participants is minimal and the potential benefits are incredible.

PROPOSAL STAGE

Over a 5-year period the idea of a nursing study with national sampling was an elusive one despite the potential significance of the study and the number of experienced researchers involved in preparing the proposal. As a collaborator/co-investigator, my role was primarily one of support—sharing potential resources, references, and writing letters.

In June 1984, I first learned of the plans for ANA's Maternal Child Health Division to develop a nursing research project with national sampling to examine nursing care needs of technology assisted children cared for at home. I was working as a clinical nurse specialist providing discharge consultation, coordinating care after discharge, and assisting in the development of models of care for ventilator-assisted youth. I volunteered to assist in any way possible after Dr. Juanita Fleming described the idea at one meeting and she notified Kathy Thomas at ANA. We discussed the project over the phone several times, and in August I sent a letter to Ms. Thomas to confirm my interest in this project.

Almost a year later, in June 1985, my résumé was requested to include with a grant proposal. At that point, my proposed role was as a member of an Advisory Council.

In July 1986, another year later, I received a letter from Dr. Fleming describing the proposed role of a liaison consultant. The idea for a national nursing study was progressing and Dr. Fleming requested written support for the study. In addition to my résumé and letter confirming my willingness to participate, information about local population numbers and access was needed.

During the next month, I contacted providers and obtained local estimates of related to technology-assisted children as well as support for this study. Although I had information about ventilator-assisted youth, I needed to know about other assistive devices for inclusion in this study. I collected information about numbers and types of agencies providing home health care, types of equipment and approximate number of children served, number of home care nurses, and number of physicians making referrals. This information, a letter of support from my employer, and a letter from a physician confirming access to the population were sent in July 1986. Dr. Fleming confirmed receipt of the information and its use in a grant proposal, and anticipated funding response by late December or early January 1987.

In October 1986, the information collected for Dr. Fleming was used to describe the Louisiana population for a pediatric home care panel presentation at the Louisiana State Nurses Association biennial convention. Panelists included a home care nurse, a home health agency administrator, and me. Participants confirmed the need, interest, and support for a national study to examine home care nursing needs of technology-assisted youth.

It was disappointing when the first submitted grant proposal for the national study was not approved. The national sampling and regional nurse researchers involved in the project were considered strengths, however. Based on the critiques of the first proposal, changes were made, circulated to collaborators/co-investigators, and resubmitted with letters indicating continued support. I simply retyped the initial letters from my employer and me using a new date.

The second grant proposal also was not approved. This time it was primarily because of costs. Telephone instead of face-to-face interviews was suggested. Resubmission with another letter of support was planned at that time. In January 1988, I sent the third set of support letters to Dr. Fleming and continued to hope that the idea for a national nursing research study would materialize.

Periodically, Dr. Fleming would call and provide an update on the status of the grant approval and funding process. In October 1989, the grant became a reality, and I began planning my participation with a new supervisor, someone who had not been involved with previous efforts. Now there was a project office, staff, and plans for a liaison consultant/collaborator/coinvestigator meeting were made. I was able to confirm my continued willingness to work on this national project and in December 1989 received the agenda and materials for a meeting in January 1990.

PREPARATION FOR THE PILOT

With approval and funding of the "High Tech" Home care grant there was a significant increase in activity. On January 13 and 14, 1990, nurses from across the country and local research consultants for the grant met in Lexington, Kentucky. The meeting was chaired by Dr. Fleming, Principal Investigator, who reviewed the history of funding for this grant and role of liaison consultant. At this time the nurses who were serving as regional representatives learned we were considered collaborators/coinvestigators. Our primary responsibilities were

1. to participate in the development of the structured interview guide;
2. to identify subjects at each site;

3. to work with agencies in obtaining subjects and send names, telephone numbers, and other pertinent information to the principal investigator or designate; and
4. to participate in the analysis and interpretation of the data. Dissemination was included with this last item.

The meeting involved incredible discussion, collaborative problem solving with some of the leading nurse researchers in the United States, and a number of small work groups. It was very well organized with some tremendous resource persons in the statisticians and telephone interview supervisor.

The draft of an interview guide was reviewed in detail. Nurses who had conducted research with this population or who were involved with clinical service [like me] had input particularly related to feasibility of items, feasibility of length of telephone interview, and family knowledge of costs. Of major concern was the sampling plan and how that could be feasible and still maintain client rights of confidentiality.

The two days of meetings were very productive. A protocol for the pilot and interview guide had been refined. The statisticians had outlined ideas for reexamining the sampling plan.

Before the end of January concerns identified during discussions were addressed and the research plan was finalized. On Monday, January 17, one of the statisticians sent me a letter to confirm some of my perceptions about the interview guide and proposed sampling scheme. Information about codes corresponding to Office of Technology Assessment stratas of technology-dependent children was requested, which I sent a week later. By return mail, the statistician sent me a letter acknowledging the hopelessness of using those codes to define group membership.

On Tuesday, January 18, Barbara Teague, the project director, sent a letter about discussions during the meeting with an abstract of study as refined, the concerns about the sampling plan, and a sample cover letter to use in contacting subjects. Postcards were to be used by subjects as the approach to release identifying information and to indicate their interest in participating in the study. The revised interview guide would be sent to collaborators/co-investigators for review when all input had been incorporated and the instrument had been piloted.

On January 30, the revised sampling scheme was sent to me. Sampling was planned in two stages, which was felt to be executable in the field and would avoid the biases that could result from a convenience sample of volunteers for study. Step 1 was to contact at most 10 home care agencies, equipment vendors, and tertiary care hospitals with pediatric home care units that care for technology-dependent children. A list of agencies, number of children in two broad categories of technology assistance, percent of children using technology on a short-term basis, and researcher/collaborator/coinvestigator comments on possible bias and sampling problems was prepared for the Kentucky statisticians and research consultants. Step 2 was the actual contact of clients through agencies selected by the Kentucky team from Step 1 information.

In less than 3 weeks the preliminary research plan had been refined with the input of the collaborators/co-investigators and the research consultants at the University of Kentucky. As a participant I found it to be an incredible experience—working with a team of nurse researchers, nurse clinicians, and support personnel a very credible research plan had been polished—and it was now time to contact agencies and finalize the sampling approach. Note that the instrument was being refined with a pilot study at the same time agency contacts were initiated in different parts of the country.

Over the next month or so I contacted all agencies in my area that provided care to technology-assisted children. I first contacted the agencies that had provided letters of support and information in mid-1986. I also contacted others in the area; some were agencies that had been opened since initial queries, and others had expanded into pediatric home care. I used my knowledge of agencies/vendors/hospitals and the Yellow Pages of the local phone book to be sure all providers had the potential to be involved. A total of 14 agencies were contacted. Four were considered not available as contact points for families, two were not providing care for children at the time, one administrator (of a for-profit home equipment company) was not comfortable with contacting clients to participate in research, and one had been providing service for a short time to a small number of short-term clients. Ten provider agencies were willing to participate, and information about their clients was sent to Kentucky for determination of sample of agencies to be approached.

Early in April 1990, I received a letter from Kentucky describing my Step 2 in the sampling plan. I was to contact 10 agencies and sample every estimated client, except with one agency who estimated 300 Group B clients; a random sampling of that subgroup was requested. To protect clients' rights, my plan was to send a letter to each potential subject family through their provider agency with a postcard for the family to return to Kentucky. No agency contacts were planned until the postcards were ready and all materials finalized for family contacts.

The report of pilot study arrived early in May 1990 with a copy of the revised interview guide and rationale for changes proposed based on pilot study. I agreed with all proposed changes and that the interview guide was feasible.

CONDUCT OF THE STUDY

Final preparations for family contacts occurred in June 1990, with plans to start agency contacts July 1, 1990. On June 6, I received salmon bifold postcards for families to return if they were interested in participating. I also received a second, regular green postcard to send to families two weeks after the initial contact letter as a reminder for them to return the salmon bifold postcard. I revised the sample contact letter to families to simplify language and to include information on how to contact me if families had questions.

Agency contacts actually started on July 5. I staggered agency contacts because I wanted to be able to schedule meetings with each agency representative and continue full-time employment. During the contacts I shared an abstract of the study and discussed options for how we could access clients to let them know about the study and determine their willingness to participate. I had packets of materials for each agency to distribute: my letter to potential subjects, a stamped salmon bifold postcard for families to return, and a business envelope and green follow-up postcard to be addressed by the agency.

During July and August, I contacted all agencies, and potential subject contacts were initiated. Three agencies accepted the packets of materials for each potential subject, added a letter from an agency representative, distributed materials to the families, and reported numbers of families contacted back to me. These were the easy ones. Five agencies scheduled meetings with me and then accepted the materials and handled them much like the first three. One agency took me out to lunch. Scheduling our meetings was sometimes difficult, but given the overall scheme this was not a major problem. A total of eight agency representatives accepted the responsibility of directly contacting subject families with prepared packets and absorbing the costs of these contacts.

A possible 150 packets were to be mailed from one agency; this was a problem. Although the agency supported the idea for this research, it could not afford the personnel time or mailing costs to contact potential subjects. I was also concerned about how to explain randomization to an agency employee so that only one-third of one group of patients would be contacted. The solution was employing a doctoral student to review the agency mailing list, randomize one group of patients, and address and stamp the envelopes and postcards to be mailed out of the agency office. Funds had been allocated in the grant to handle such problems. This was not complicated but did require more time and expense than other potential subject contacts had required.

A total of nine agencies were used to contact potential subjects. The tenth, a branch of a national firm, was deleted because scheduling the meeting with the local administrator was difficult and still had not been done when an adequate sample from this region had been obtained.

There were some concerns identified during the agency contacts of potential subjects that needed to be addressed. Initially, I had been concerned that the estimated and actual numbers of clients were different; however, this balanced out in the long run. One agency was a branch of a national company, and its administration required more specific information about the national study before the local agency could distribute packets to clients. One agency had clients who were out of state, actually in another collaborator's/coinvestigator's area, and we had to be sure this client could be a subject. This problem had been addressed during research planning stages with color-coding of client postcards so that the Kentucky researchers would be able to track how the clients learned about the study. One agency administrator was a nursing master's degree student and needed to review the complete protocol—this occurred only once during all my agency contacts. One agency had a number of clients with little formal education and no telephone, and their nurses were concerned that few clients would return the postcards. That agency decided to have individual home health nurses describe the study to families and, if families were interested in participating, assist the family when it filled out the identifying information on the salmon postcard. I was impressed with these nurses and their commitment to promoting the involvement of their clients in such a research study.

CONCLUSION

This had been an incredible experience. With a principal investigator and research team in Kentucky, I have been able to participate in a national research study with minimal expenditure of time. Many of the onerous details of research were not problems, and I was able to concentrate on the fun parts—developing instruments, contacting subjects, reviewing re-sults, and providing input into analysis.

As early as August 1990, 33 families from my area had responded, and that number grew to 93 by December. Given the expertise and energy that has gone into the planning and implementation of this national study, I believe my region was well represented in the national study. This popula-tion had a voice in results presented to policymakers as well as caregivers with the potential to affect the support and services for technology-assisted youth and their families.

I hope other nurse researchers can be encouraged by this process. Research can be incorporated into clinical activities. By working with a team, a larger population can be accessed and validity concerns minimized. It does require some time, but with a commitment to research, it's definitely worthwhile, and we can all contribute to the knowledge base for nursing.

Index